牙体牙髓病学 PBL 教学案例集

（学生版）

PBL Cases of Cariology and Endodontics

(Student Edition)

江千舟　主　编

曾素娟　杨　莉　副主编

北方联合出版传媒（集团）股份有限公司

辽宁科学技术出版社

沈　阳

图文编辑

杨　帆　刘　娜　张　浩　刘玉卿　肖　艳　刘　菲　康　鹤　王静雅　纪凤薇　杨　洋

图书在版编目（CIP）数据

牙体牙髓病学PBL教学案例集：学生版/江千舟主编.—沈阳：辽宁科学技术出版社，2022.10
ISBN 978-7-5591-2689-4

Ⅰ．①牙…　Ⅱ．①江…　Ⅲ．①牙髓病－医案－汇编　Ⅳ.①R781.3

中国版本图书馆CIP数据核字（2022）第151923号

出版发行：辽宁科学技术出版社
　　　　　（地址：沈阳市和平区十一纬路25号　邮编：110003）
印 刷 者：辽宁一诺广告印务有限公司
经 销 者：各地新华书店
幅面尺寸：210mm×285mm
印　　张：9
字　　数：180千字
出版时间：2022年10月第1版
印刷时间：2022年10月第1次印刷
策划编辑：陈　刚
责任编辑：杨晓宇
封面设计：盼　盼
版式设计：盼　盼
责任校对：李　霞

书　　号：ISBN 978-7-5591-2689-4
定　　价：98.00元

投稿热线：024-23280336
邮购热线：024-23280336
E-mail:cyclonechen@126.com
http://www.lnkj.com.cn

编委会

主 编

江千舟

副主编

曾素娟　杨　莉

编 者

何　颖　黄雨婷　闫　亮　王一舟　李益玲
张文娟　赵　健　刘　晓　孔媛媛　涂欣冉
蔡冬萍　吴　磊　方　颖　封　琼　盛　婷

译 者

徐静怡　陈荣丰　刘珍妮　温思怡　谭国忠
梁梓添　陈　彦

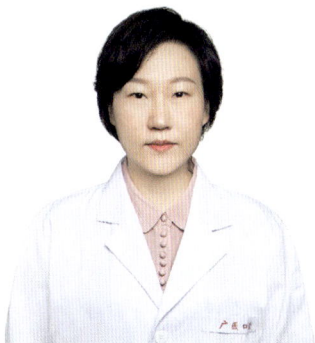

江千舟

口腔医学博士、博士研究生导师
广州医科大学口腔医学院牙体牙髓病学教研室主任
广州医科大学附属口腔医院牙体牙髓科主任、教学管理科主任

　　1997年本科毕业于湖北医科大学口腔医学院（现武汉大学口腔医学院）口腔医学专业，后取得武汉大学口腔医学博士学位。现任中华口腔医学会牙体牙髓病学专业委员会常务委员、中华口腔医学会老年口腔医学专业委员会委员、广东省口腔医学会口腔医学教育专业委员会副主任委员、广东省口腔医学会牙体牙髓病学专业委员会副主任委员、广东省女医师协会口腔分会副主任委员、广东省口腔医学会理事、广东省口腔医师协会理事。《Oral Diseases》《Journal of Periodontology》《Microscopy Research and Technique》等杂志特约审稿人。

　　从事教学、医疗、科研工作20余年，多年来负责或参与牙体牙髓病学、口腔医学导论、口腔预防医学、口腔专业外语等理论和实践教学。作为课程负责人，所负责的"牙体牙髓病学"获批省级精品课程、省级线上线下混合式一流课程。培养研究生20余名，主持或参加多项国家、省部级课题，发表相关科研学术论文80余篇，其中SCI收录30余篇。主编专著3部、参编专著2部。擅长牙体牙髓疾病的诊治。

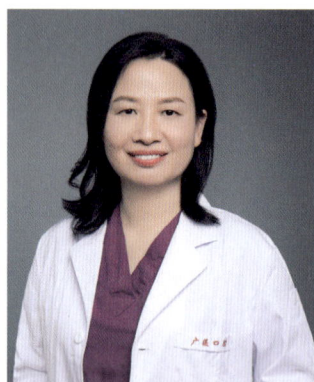

曾素娟

医学博士、硕士研究生导师

广州医科大学口腔医学院儿童口腔医学教研室主任

广州医科大学附属口腔医院儿童口腔科主任

　　1994年本科毕业于湖南医科大学（现中南大学湘雅口腔医学院）口腔医学专业，后取得中山大学口腔临床医学硕士学位、南方医科大学临床医学博士学位。现任中华口腔医学会儿童口腔医学专业委员会常务委员、广东省口腔医学会儿童口腔医学专业委员会副主任委员、广东省口腔医学会镇静镇痛专业委员会副主任委员。《实用医学杂志》审稿专家。

　　从事教学、医疗、科研工作20余年，多年来负责或参与儿童口腔医学、口腔预防医学、牙体牙髓病学、口腔医学导论等理论和实践教学。主编《儿童牙外伤诊疗图解》，参编国家卫生健康委员会"十三五"规划教材、全国高等学校教材《口腔科学》。发表论文50余篇。主持或参与各级课题10余项。擅长全身麻醉下儿童口腔疾病的治疗、儿童龋病的综合防治、乳牙及年轻恒牙的牙髓根尖周病诊疗、儿童牙外伤的诊治、儿童错殆畸形的早期矫治、牙齿发育异常的诊治等。

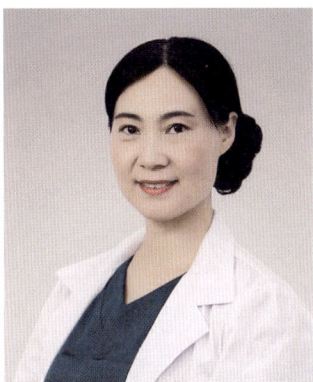

杨莉

主任医师

硕士研究生导师

广州医科大学附属口腔医院东晓南门诊部主任

　　1993年毕业于湖北医科大学口腔医学院（现武汉大学口腔医学院）口腔医学专业。第四届"羊城好医生"。现任广东省口腔医学会老年口腔医学专业委员会副主任委员、广东省口腔医学会牙体牙髓病学专业委员会常务委员、广东省口腔医学会儿童口腔医学专业委员会常务委员，广州医科大学附属口腔医院住院医师规范化培训口腔全科基地负责人。长期从事口腔临床、保健、教学、科研工作。主编专著1部、参编专著2部。主持完成省级课题3项。发表科研论文30余篇。

　　数千年来，传统的中国教学模式是以学科和教师为中心的教学模式，基本上是教师讲、学生听。这种教学模式可将教师的积极性发挥到极致，但这是一种"灌输式"的教学模式，学生多数是通过死记硬背学习知识，而主观能动性发挥不足。这类缺陷具有普遍性，古今中外的教育中均有所存在。为了克服这类缺陷和偏向，PBL教学模式应运而生。所谓PBL教学模式是以问题为导向（Problem-Based Learning）的，于1969年由美国神经病学教授Barrows在加拿大McMaster大学医学院正式推出，此后美国及欧洲、亚洲等国家的医学院校先后效仿。目前，国际上已有1700余所医学院校采用这种教学模式进行教学。

　　PBL教学模式有以下特征：让学生成为情景中的角色，这样可以使学生全神贯注、思想集中、积极参与；教师围绕这一具体问题设计、安排课程，鼓励学生动脑筋思考，并追溯相关问题和知识，拓宽学生的知识面，不断引导学生深入理解问题；PBL教学过程是真实情景再现，学生发挥积极性、主动性和创造性，对复杂的医学问题进行深度学习与思考。

　　PBL教学模式过程首先应包括准备过程，需要教师讲解总论和概论以作为课程的过渡；然后由学生提出问题，进行小组讨论，集思广益，在讨论中相互补充、相互启发；最后再进行课堂大讨论，将问题集中、总结。学习过程中以学生为主体，教师仅起到辅助作用。

　　很多学者会问：为什么PBL教学模式会在医学院开始推广？这是医学固有的属性使然。第一，医学院的学生将来面对的是患者，单纯的背书是不够的，必须能够讲解明白，使患者能理解患病原因及相关知识；第二，每名患者的疾病不尽相同，需要独立思考、分析，医生需要全面了解病情，全程参与；第三，医学是一门不断发展、变化的学科，医学知识不断更新，学生要不断学习、终身学习，才能满足临床需要；第四，医学也是一门社会科学，单掌握医疗技术是远远不够的，还需要具有沟通能力，医生需要在实践中锻炼、提高，能够融会贯通地给患者讲解。PBL教学模式正是这样一种良好的学习手段。PBL教学模式是以学生为主体、基于问题的教学模式。在指导教师的参与下，学生以小组为单位，基于复杂的病例提出问题、进行讨论。在这一过程中，学生是课堂的主体，教师仅起到辅助作用。由教师帮助学生，让学生在学习过程中主动学习知识，这样学到的知识特别牢固，并且记忆深刻。

　　广州医科大学口腔医学院比较早地就开始探索PBL教学实践，开展国际学术交流，派遣一些优秀教授赴国外参观、交流、学习，具有比较丰富的教学经验，所以编写此书具有一定基础。

  本书内容仅涉及龋病、牙髓病和根尖周病以及牙体硬组织非龋性疾病，没有包含口腔学科的全部内容。但是，这一部分内容特别适合采用PBL教学模式。广义地说，这些内容都属于口腔内科学范畴，由于口腔内科学的学习内容比较精细，小组讨论方式比较直观，可以详细了解局部解剖，指导精细操作，使学生成为合格的牙体牙髓科医生，最后成为牙体牙髓专科医生。

  本书为学生的学习创造了一个良好的机会，希望大家珍惜这些被教师辛苦摸索出来的经验，充分利用好本书，预祝大家成为一名合格的牙体牙髓科医生。

武汉大学口腔医学院

2022年5月

以问题为导向（Problem–Based Learning，PBL）的教学模式，是以学生为中心的教育方式。与传统的以学科为基础的教学模式有很大不同，PBL教学强调以学生的主动学习为主，而不是以传统教学中的教师讲课为主。PBL教学模式非常贴合临床医学教学特点，教学中以临床病例为先导，以问题为基础，以学生为主体，在教师引导下进行启发式教育，更贴近临床实际，有益于培养医学生临床诊治能力。PBL教学也是口腔医学临床实习教学改革的重要内容。

广州医科大学口腔医学院已开展PBL教学多年，在教学经验积累的基础上组织编写了这本《牙体牙髓病学PBL教学案例集（学生版）》。我看到这本书后，感觉广州医科大学口腔医学院牙体牙髓病学同仁在PBL教学方面走在了国内同行的前列，这是一本非常实用的好书。有两个特点：首先，确定了每节课的教学目标，明确了学生需掌握、熟悉和了解的问题；其次，"课程思政"部分也是我在国内教科书中第一次见到，将思政教育贯穿于教学始终，对于培养有爱心和责任心的医生非常重要。本书中"课程设计"和"案例简介"内容丰富，紧密结合临床。启发式教育有益于培养学生独立学习和思考能力。本书还有一大特点是用中文和英文书写，对于提高学生的双语能力、发展国际视野，是非常有意义的。

本书的出版对于促进国内口腔医学院校教育推广PBL教学，培养适合临床需要的口腔医学人才是很有益的。真诚地希望广州医科大学口腔医学院的编写团队——主编江千舟教授和副主编曾素娟教授、杨莉教授，不断总结PBL教学经验，奉献给同仁。

北京大学口腔医学院

葛立宏

2022年5月8日于北京

在国际竞争日趋激烈的21世纪，高等教育扮演着越来越重要的角色。各个国家都在采取各种措施进行高等教育改革，按照《中国教育现代化2035》精神，国内各大院校都在积极进行教学改革和教学模式的探索来提高本科教育的质量。传统的教学模式以教师讲授为主，学生被动接受"灌输式"知识，学习效果不理想，尤其对于口腔医学实践技能要求较高的学科来说更加突出。

牙体牙髓病学是一门口腔临床专业主干学科，是口腔医学的重要组成部分。学生主要学习牙体牙髓病学的基本理论知识，并针对牙体牙髓疾病的预防、诊断、治疗等方面进行临床实践，要求学生掌握诊断、治疗相关疾病，并具备预防保健的应用能力。结合牙体牙髓病学的特点，我们于2011年开始探索"以问题为导向（Problem-Based Learning，PBL）"的教学模式，并借鉴荷兰奈梅亨牙学院自主学习（Self-Study Assignment，SSA）的教学方式，进行了有益的尝试，取得了一定的经验。课程安排是在理论课的基础上增设PBL教学，指导学生自主学习，发现问题、提出问题，将传统的以"教师讲授为主"的模式转向"学生自主"学习，将学习的决定权从教师转移给学生，提高学生自主学习的兴趣和能力，锻炼学生独立思考的能力，充分提升学生在学习过程中的自主性、积极性、互动性和创造性，从而优化教学质量和提升学习效果，以培养学生的自学能力、实践能力、团队合作精神。

PBL教学是由8～10名学生和1名教师组成的讨论小组，围绕某一具体病例的疾病诊治等问题进行讨论，为满足教学的同质化，我们将前期的经验成果编写成这本《牙体牙髓病学PBL教学案例集（学生版）》，精选了有代表性的临床案例场景14个，覆盖牙体牙髓病学研究的主要疾病，适用于口腔专业的学生使用。

据WHO报告，全球目前约有1700所医学院采用PBL教学模式，而这个数字还在不断增加，在我国也有多所院校的医学教育工作者在某些医学课程的教学中应用或借鉴了PBL教学模式，《牙体牙髓病学PBL教学案例集》包括两个部分——学生版和教师版。由于时间紧，编者水平有限，存在不当或疏漏之处，诚恳各位教师和学生批评指正，以便再版时修改。

广州医科大学口腔医学院

2022年6月

第一章
龋病

第一节　"小黑点"成长记

教学目标

掌握

1. 龋病病因的四联因素学说理论。

2. 浅龋、中龋的临床表现，诊断方法和诊断标准。

3. 龋病非手术治疗的方法。

熟悉

1. 与龋病发病关系密切的微生物及其致龋特征。

2. 龋病的临床分类。

3. 龋病风险评估与不同龋病风险等级的管理。

了解

1. 龋病的概念、流行情况，龋病流行病学指标和调查方法。

2. 牙菌斑生物膜的形成过程。

3. 龋病的病理过程。

4. 龋病综合治疗的理念，常用的龋病风险评估表。

能力目标

引导学生完成学习目标时要注重理论联系实际，为龋病临床诊断打好基础，培养临床思辨能力。鼓励学生进行龋病病因的探索，分析龋病过程中牙齿的修复和基本病理变化，激发学生对龋病生物治疗方法的研究兴趣。

1

课程思政

1. 了解全球龋病发病状况，结合病例，培养学生良好的口腔卫生习惯，增强学生对国内口腔疾病防治的使命感。分析龋病病因的四联因素，鼓励学生进行龋病病因的探索。

2. 结合病例，培养学生对疾病发病的关注，引入人文关怀，增强学生作为口腔医生的责任感，向学生倡导以患者为中心、医者仁心的重要性。

3. 结合健康全生命周期管理理念，培养学生对疾病预防及治疗的关注，增强人民生命全周期健康服务的意识。

课程设计

1. 课前学生8～10人为1组，阅读案例后提出问题，以问题为导向的方式列出学习重点，查找资料，课前文献阅读4学时（每学时40分钟），课上案例讨论2学时（其中脑力激荡10分钟、问题列举5分钟、讨论及引导50分钟、总结15分钟）。以龋病的定义、龋病的好发牙位与好发牙面、牙菌斑的形成与发育、牙菌斑微生物学与致龋性、龋病病因学的现代概念、龋病的发病机制等为学习目标。需要掌握的内容讨论时间占80%，需要熟悉及了解的内容讨论时间占20%。

2. 课后作业：讨论结束后每人需交1篇小组讨论记录并完成课后作业，包括讨论时遇到的问题，查找、组织材料时遇到的困难。

3. 评价方式：课上表现占70%，作业占30%。课上表现使用自评、组内及组间互评、教师评价表评分（教师评价包括纪律性、参与度、组内影响力、团队合作力、协调能力等方面）。

案例简介

本案例学习浅龋、中龋相关内容，设计分为两幕进行。

第一幕通过临床问诊引导学生学习龋病的定义、牙菌斑的形成、牙菌斑微生物学、常见的致龋微生物、微生物与龋病之间的关系、牙菌斑的物质代谢、牙菌斑的致龋过程。帮助学生学习并掌握龋病四联因素学说理论。

第二幕提供临床案例的口内照，表现龋病发生不同阶段的临床特点，让学生对龋病进行分类，提出检查方法并对龋病进行诊断；重点让学生掌握龋病的分类、临床表现及诊断标准。

关键词

牙菌斑，微生物，矿化，四联因素学说理论，浅龋，中龋，急性龋，慢性龋，继发龋

第一幕

　　23岁的崔先生来口腔医院看病，挂了张医生的专家号，在诊室外候诊，护士在询问崔先生的病情及病史后让其等待。

　　10分钟后，崔先生坐在治疗椅上。

　　崔先生对张医生说："我很多颗牙齿都莫名其妙地黄一块、缺一块，已经有1年多了。"

　　张医生说："那让我看看你的牙齿，是不是像你所说的那样。"

　　崔先生立刻紧张起来，一旁的护士安慰他："我们现在只是检查一下，并不会有什么不舒服的感觉。放松，放心，张医生会轻轻地给你检查。"

　　张医生在看到口腔内的情况后，发现患者的牙周和牙齿状况确实比较差，在临床中这种情况多发生于年轻患者，但不是很常见。

　　口腔内检查结果：全口卫生较差，牙间隙存在大量食物残渣及软垢；牙龈红肿，探诊出血；14、24、34、31、41、44牙颈部龋坏和着色，其中14、24、34在牙颈部龋坏的冠方可见白垩色斑块样物质；12、11、21、22、23、33、42、43有充填物，边缘着色（图1）。

　　崔先生在检查中焦急地问："张医生，我的牙齿情况糟糕吗？能不能治好？"

　　张医生在检查后说："可以治疗，但是龋坏的牙齿较多，并且之前补过的牙齿又开始烂了，比较复杂。你之前有做过其他治疗吗？"

　　崔先生回答："做过根管治疗，但那是在麻醉后做的。上次补牙时磨牙很酸，就补了几个。"

　　张医生对崔先生说："你需要补的牙齿有很多，并且有些牙齿是需要重新补的，如果牙齿敏感度较高，在补牙时需要局部麻醉。"

　　崔先生问张医生："为什么牙齿坏了这么多？我天天刷牙，为什么牙齿的状况还这么差？我又不吸烟，牙齿颜色还这么黄，是不是我的口腔里有较多的虫？"

　　张医生说："龋坏不是虫，是细菌等因素共同作用所形成的牙齿组织缺损。你是做什么工作的？一天工作多久？有没有熬夜的习惯？"

　　崔先生回答："这有什么关系吗？我的工作是图纸设计。熬夜是经常的。我比较喜欢喝可乐，渴了也不喝水，而是喝可乐。"

张医生惊讶地问："那你一天要喝多少？"

崔先生回答："差不多六七瓶吧。"

张医生觉得补牙是必需的，但是如果崔先生不改变饮食习惯，即使牙齿被补好了也还会继续发生龋坏。所以，必须要让患者知道，其饮食习惯对牙齿造成了很大的影响。而且患者的牙周情况较差，对补牙有着较大的影响。在进行口腔卫生宣教及龋病常识普及后，建议崔先生先进行牙周治疗，等牙周恢复正常后再进行补牙。

崔先生同意了治疗方案，预约了后期补牙。

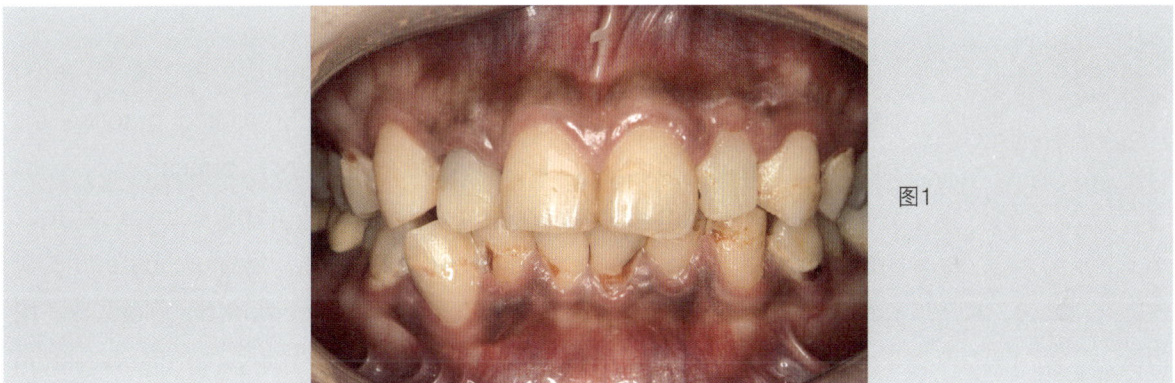

图1

患者资料	拟实施治疗计划
推断 / 假设	拟学习的问题

Act I

Mr. Cui, 23 years old, made an appointment with Dr. Zhang. In the waiting room, the nurse asked him about his condition and medical history.

Ten minutes later, Mr. Cui sat in the dental chair.

"There is no reason that most of my teeth have turned yellow and been defected for over a year." Mr. Cui said.

"Let me see if your teeth are as you described." Dr. Zhang said.

Mr. Cui immediately got nervous and the nurse on the side reassured him and said, "Take it easy. We are just taking a medical check and there won't be any discomfort. Just relax and Dr. Zhang will give you a gentle check."

After checking the situation, Dr. Zhang found that the patient's periodontal and tooth condition was indeed poor. In clinical practice, this situation mostly occurs in young patients, but it is not common.

Intraoral examination: poor general oral hygiene with great food impaction in the interspace; gingiva is red and swollen, bleeding on probing; 14, 24, 34, 31, 41 and 44 cervical caries and discoloration; 12, 11, 21, 22, 23, 33, 42 and 43 with fillings and marginal discoloration; 14, 24 and 34 with chalky plaque-like material on the coronal side of the cervical caries (Figure 1).

Mr. Cui asked anxiously during the examination, "Dr. Zhang, is my tooth in bad condition? Can it be cured?"

After the examination, Dr. Zhang replied, "It can be treated, but there are a great number of decayed teeth and the teeth filled previously have begun to decay again, which is more complicated. Have you done any other treatment before?"

"I have had root canal therapy under anesthesia. I felt sore greatly during tooth filling, so I just finished several." Mr. Cui replied.

"You need to fill a lot of teeth, and some of them need to be refilled. If your teeth are sensitive to the treatment, anesthesia is required during tooth filling." Dr. Zhang said.

Mr. Cui asked Dr. Zhang, "Why do I have so much tooth decay? I brush my teeth every day, but they are still in such bad condition. I don't smoke, but my teeth are still yellow. Are there any worms in my mouth?"

"Worms? Caries is not a worm. It is a kind of tooth defect caused by germs and other factors. What do you do? How long do you work per day? Do you get used to staying up late?" Dr. Zhang asked.

"Does it matter? I work as a drawing designer. And it's common to stay up late. I prefer to drink Coke instead of water." Mr. Cui said.

Dr. Zhang asked surprisingly, "Then how much do you drink a day?"

"About 6 or 7 bottles." Mr. Cui answered.

Dr. Zhang believed that the filling was necessary, but if Mr. Cui could not change his eating habits, dental caries would continue to occur even after the filling. So it was important to let the patient know that his eating habits had a great impact on his teeth. And the patient's poor periodontal condition had a great impact on the filling. It was recommended that Mr. Cui should finish the periodontal treatment first and start the filling after the periodontal tissue has returned to normal. Mr. Cui agreed to the treatment plan, went for periodontal treatment and made an appointment for the later filling.

Patient information	Actions to take
Inference/Assumption	Question to study

第二幕

2周后，崔先生的牙周状况有了明显改善，学会了正确刷牙和控制牙菌斑的方法。按照预约好的时间来到张医生的诊室。

张医生对14、24、34、31、41、44进行了去腐、备洞、树脂充填；对14、24、34白垩色斑块处进行渗透树脂治疗；对12、11、21、22、23、33、42、43进行去除充填物边缘的龋坏、备洞、树脂充填。

患者资料	拟实施治疗计划
推断 / 假设	拟学习的问题

Act II

Two weeks later, Mr. Cui's periodontal condition had improved greatly, and he had learned how to brush and control the dental plaque properly. He came to Dr. Zhang's clinic at the appointed time.

Dr. Zhang performed decay removal, cavity preparation, and resin filling on 14, 24, 34, 31, 41 and 44; resin infiltration treatment on chalky plaques on 14, 24 and 34; and decay filling removal, cavity preparation and resin filling on 12, 11, 21, 22, 23, 33, 42 and 43.

Patient information	Actions to take
Inference/Assumption	Question to study

编者：何　颖　黄雨婷

译者：徐静怡

第二节　小小"黑点"，别有洞天

教学目标

掌握

1. 深龋的临床表现、诊断方法及诊断标准。

2. 牙釉质和牙髓牙本质复合体的生物学基础。

3. 牙体修复与材料选择的原则。

4. 深龋治疗的原则及盖髓术的适应证。

熟悉

1. 龋病的临床分类，龋病风险评估与不同龋病风险等级的管理措施。

2. 复合树脂的分类、性能与临床应用。

3. 间接盖髓术和直接盖髓术的操作步骤。

了解

1. 龋病综合治疗的理念。

2. 常用龋病风险评估表。

3. 牙体粘接材料的发展过程。

能力目标

在第一节的学习基础上加深对深龋的理解，掌握龋病非手术治疗方法的种类、各种治疗方法的特点以及牙体修复材料的选择，培养临床思辨能力。分析龋病早期治疗及深龋发生过程中牙齿的修复，鼓励学生进行龋病预防及治疗方法的探索研究。

课程思政

1. 了解龋病的危险因素，结合龋病预防措施，培养学生树立健康全生命周期管理理念，增强学生对国内口腔疾病防治的使命感。

2. 结合健康全生命周期管理理念，培养学生对疾病预防及治疗的关注，分析龋病的危险因素，鼓励学生进行龋病预防的探索。

课程设计

1. 课前学生8~10人为1组，阅读案例后提出问题，以问题为导向列出学习重点，查找资料，课前文献阅读4学时，课上案例讨论2学时（其中脑力激荡10分钟、问题列举5分钟、讨论及引导50分钟、总结15分钟）。以深龋的临床表现、诊断方法及诊断标准；牙釉质和牙髓牙本质复合体的生物学基础；牙体修复与材料选择的原则等为学习目标。需要掌握的内容讨论时间占80%，需要熟悉及了解的内容讨论时间占20%。

2. 课后作业：讨论结束后每人需交1篇小组讨论记录并完成课后作业，包括讨论时遇到的问题，查找、组织材料时遇到的困难。

3. 评价方式：课上表现占70%、作业占30%。课上表现使用自评、组内及组间互评、教师评价表评分（教师评价包括纪律性、参与度、组内影响力、团队合作力、协调能力等方面）。

案例简介

本案例学习深龋相关内容，设计分为两幕进行。

第一幕主要讨论深龋的临床表现、诊断方法及诊断标准；牙釉质和牙髓牙本质复合体的生物学基础；牙体修复治疗术的定义、修复方法与材料选择的原则；窝洞预备的基本原则及步骤；深龋治疗的原则及盖髓术的适应证。希望学生学习并掌握深龋的临床表现及特点，同时提供相关参考文献，指导学生对深龋临床特点的理解。

第二幕主要讨论粘接系统及树脂粘接修复，与临床结合较紧密。主要内容有酸蚀刻技术、玷污层、酸蚀-冲洗粘接系统、自酸蚀粘接系统的概念；牙釉质、牙本质的粘接机制；牙本质粘接系统的分类和临床选择；复合树脂粘接修复术的适应证、禁忌证、优缺点和临床操作步骤。同时提供临床案例的口内照，让学生对深龋有进一步的理解。

关键词

深龋，牙髓牙本质复合体，增龄性变化，修复性反应，窝洞预备，粘接

第一幕

23岁的小林来口腔医院看病，挂了何医生的号，在诊室外候诊，护士在询问小林病情及病史后让其等待。

10分钟后，护士将小林安排在何医生的治疗椅上。

何医生："你哪里不舒服？"

小林："喝冷水时我的左下后牙有点儿痛，已经有一段时间了，尤其是早上刷牙的时候比较明显，但是过一会儿又不痛了，如果再喝冷的就又有点儿痛了。"

何医生："晚上会痛吗？不接触冷水的时候痛吗？"

小林："其他时候没有什么感觉，只是接触冷水时特别明显。"

何医生："让我检查一下你的牙齿，看看出了什么问题。"

小林看到何医生拿的探针立刻紧张起来："这么尖的工具，会不会很痛啊？"一旁的护士安慰小林："不会的，我们现在只是检查一下，很轻的，看看是哪颗牙齿出了问题。"

何医生也安慰小林，首先看了一下口腔内的情况，接着用探针仔细进行了检查。

口腔内检查结果：全口卫生状况一般，牙龈未见明显红肿，探诊不出血；37探及深龋洞，内有大量食物残渣、探诊酸软；36𬌗面见白色充填物，边缘继发龋坏，探诊时可钩住探针，无探痛（图2）。

小林："何医生，我的牙齿情况怎么样？"

何医生："你的牙齿烂得比较多哦，并且左下牙烂得有点儿深，我探查这颗牙的时候你都有感觉了，对吗？"

小林："是的，我就感觉左下的牙齿有问题，但无法确定是哪颗，问题严重吗？是补一下就行，还是需要做根管治疗？"

何医生："看来你对治疗有一定了解，现在无法完全判定是哪颗牙齿让您不舒服，龋坏的牙齿比较多，还需做进一步检查。"

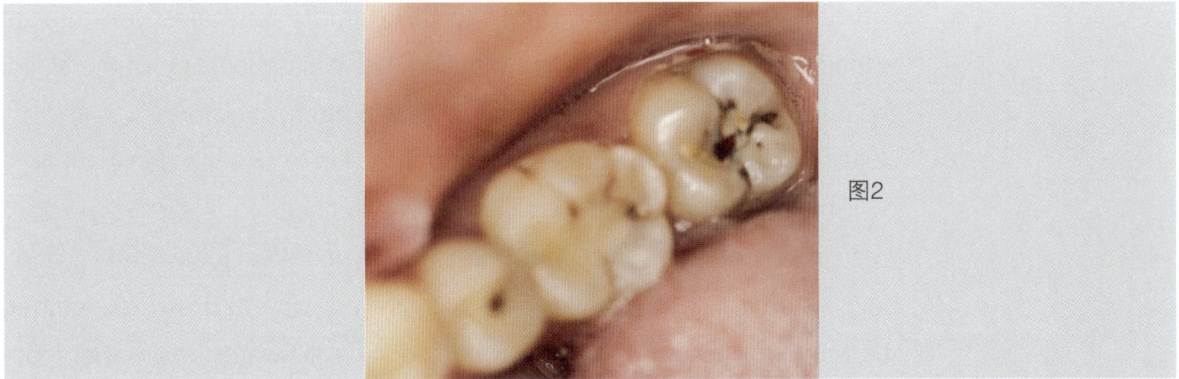

图2

患者资料	拟实施治疗计划
推断 / 假设	拟学习的问题

Act Ⅰ

Xiao Lin, 23 years old, came to the dental hospital and made an appointment with Dr. He. When Xiao Lin was waiting outside of the clinic, the nurse asked him about his condition and medical history.

Ten minutes later, the nurse assigned Xiao Lin to Dr. He's dental chair.

"What are you not feeling well and how can I help you?" Dr. He asked.

"I get a toothache in my left mandibular posterior tooth when I drink cold water. It's been a while, especially severe when I brush my teeth in the morning, but I feel better later. If I drink cold water again, that tooth hurts a bit again." Xiao Lin answered.

"Do you feel painful at night? Does it hurt when you don't drink the cold water?" Dr. He asked.

"I feel nothing. Only when I drink cold water, the pain is obvious." Xiao Lin answered.

"Let me check your teeth to see what's wrong." Dr. He said.

Xiao Lin immediately became nervous when he saw the probe tip that Dr. He was holding, "Such a sharp tool, will it hurt?" The nurse placated him, "Take it easy. We're just checking now. It's very gentle. Let's see which tooth has the problem."

Dr. He also reassured Xiao Lin. Firstly, Dr. He took a look at the general situation in his mouth, and then carefully examined it with a probe.

Intraoral examination shows that the oral hygiene is not bad, with no obvious redness or swelling of the gingiva, no bleeding on probing; 37, deep cavities with a large amount of food residue, feeling sore during exploration probing; 36, white filling on the occlusal surface, secondary caries on its margin (Figure 2).

"Dr. He, how are my teeth?" Xiao Lin asked.

"Your teeth decayed a lot, and your left mandibular posterior tooth got deep caries. You could feel it when I probed it, right?" Dr. He said.

"Yes, I felt something was wrong with the left mandibular tooth, but I can't tell which one it is. Is it serious? Is it enough to fill it up or do I need root canal therapy?" Xiao Lin asked.

"You know quite a lot. I can't determine which tooth makes you uncomfortable because you have so many decayed teeth. So I need to carry out further examinations." Dr. He said.

Patient information	Actions to take
Inference/Assumption	Question to study

第二幕

何医生对患者的口腔进行进一步全面检查。

何医生："首先，我需要给这个区域的牙齿做个冷热测试，再去拍一张牙片来确定牙齿龋坏的程度，根据这些检查的结果来决定做什么治疗。有的牙齿需要做充填修复，有的也许要做根管治疗，治疗过程中如果牙齿敏感度较高，我们会用一点麻药，不会让你感觉到痛的。"

小林有点害羞地说："我来医院前在网上查了一下，网上也是说像我这种情况，有的需要补牙，有的要做根管治疗。那就按照您说的做吧。"

何医生："好的，我们先做冷热测试，根据测试结果先判断你的牙齿状态，再根据牙片来综合判断你酸痛的牙齿是哪颗？"

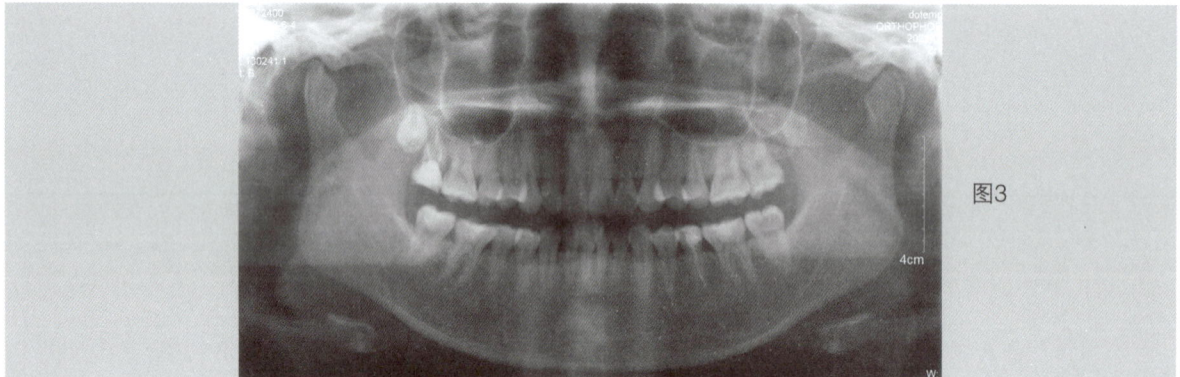

图3

小林做完一系列检查（图3）后回到诊室："何医生，到底是哪颗牙齿出了问题？严重吗？"

何医生："初步判断是左下第七颗牙齿引起的酸痛，但是要去除龋坏的牙体组织后才能判断龋坏的程度。"

小林："好的，那就尽快治疗吧。"

何医生去除龋坏时发现37龋坏较深，引起疼痛，36有继发龋坏，建议小林进行充填治疗，并详细解释了治疗相关事宜，小林同意了治疗方案。于是何医生给患牙上了橡皮障，轻轻去除龋坏牙体组织，将37用树脂材料进行充填（图4），并预约对其他牙齿进行处理。

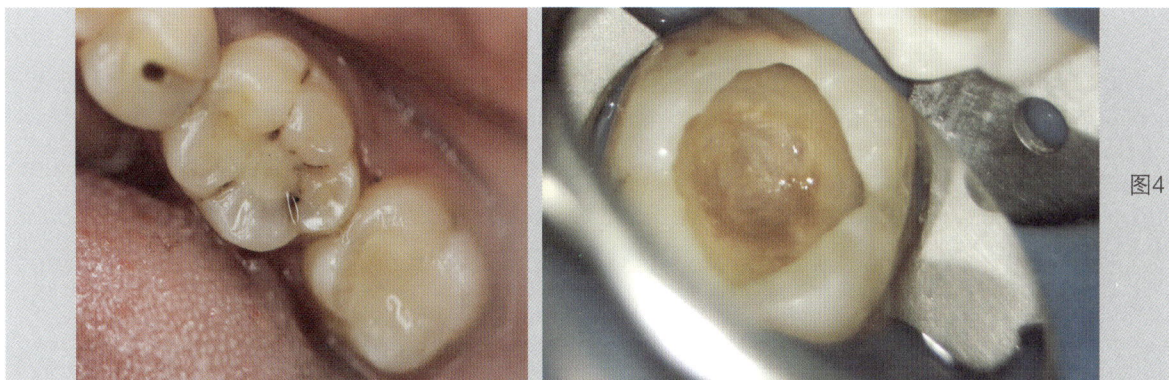

图4

患者资料	拟实施治疗计划
推断 / 假设	拟学习的问题

Act II

Dr. He performed a thorough oral examination on the patient.

"Firstly, I need to test the tooth in this area and then take the radiographic examination to determine the extent of the tooth decay. I will make a treatment plan depending the results of these tests. Some teeth will need to be filled and restored, and maybe some will need root canal therapy. If the tooth is highly sensitive during the treatment, we will use a little anesthesia to make you feel less painful." Dr. He said.

"I searched online before I came to the hospital. It's also said that in my case, some teeth need to be filled and some need root canal therapy. Just do as you say." Xiao Lin said.

"OK, let's do the hot and cold test first. Based on the test results, we'll first judge the condition of your teeth. Then according to the results of the radiographic examination, we will determine which tooth is causing the soreness." Dr. He said.

Xiao Lin returned to the clinic after a series of tests (Figure 3) and asked, "Dr. He, which tooth has the problem? Is it serious?"

"The initial judgment is that it's the last mandibular molar that causes the soreness, but the degree of the decay can only be determined after removing the decayed tooth tissue. Don't worry." Dr. He answered.

"OK, then let's do the treatment as soon as possible." Xiao Lin answered.

Dr. He removed the decay and found the painful mandibular left seventh tooth was deeply decayed and the mandibular left sixth tooth had secondary decay, so he suggested Xiao Lin take the filling treatment and explained the treatment in detail. Xiao Lin agreed to the treatment plan. Dr. He then placed a rubber dam on the affected tooth, removed the decayed tissue gently, filled the decayed mandibular left seventh tooth with a resin material (Figure 4), and made an appointment to treat other teeth next time.

Patient information	Actions to take
Inference/Assumption	Question to study

编者：闫 亮 何 颖

译者：徐静怡

第三节　推广普及龋病的早期预防

教学目标

掌握
1. 牙菌斑的控制在龋病预防中的作用。
2. 龋病的三级预防。
3. 氟化物防龋机制。
4. 窝沟封闭的临床应用（适应证、操作步骤、注意事项）。
5. 氟化物的全身和局部应用（原理、方法、剂量、优缺点等）。
6. 预防性树脂充填（适应证、操作步骤）。
7. 非创伤性修复治疗（适应证、操作步骤）。
8. 渗透树脂治疗（适应证、操作步骤）。

熟悉
1. 龋病病因。
2. 氟牙症的诊断和分类（Dean标准）。

了解
1. 激光、免疫以及替代性预防的基本概念。
2. 氟的适宜摄入量、中毒量和致死量。
3. 窝沟龋的预防方法及评估。

能力目标
学习并掌握龋病预防的方法、适应证、优缺点及操作步骤，熟悉龋病病因。通过文献的阅读，掌握口腔专业英语词汇。了解提出问题–查阅资料–解决问题的自学方法。

课程思政

通过讨论目前国内的龋病患病状况及医疗卫生条件，加强作为口腔医务工作者的责任感，加强健康宣教，提升口腔健康水平，降低龋病发病率。

课程设计

1. 课前学生8~10人为1组分配任务，阅读案例后提出问题，以问题为导向列出学习重点，查找资料，课前文献阅读4学时，课上案例讨论2学时（其中脑力激荡10分钟、问题列举5分钟、讨论及引导50分钟、总结15分钟）。

2. 课后作业：预习并准备第二幕讨论，准备5分钟小情景剧，表演水平颤动拂刷法的指导，指导者由第二次课上教师抽签决定。

3. 评价方式：课上表现占70%，作业占30%。课上表现使用自评、组内及组间互评、教师评价表评分（教师评价包括纪律性、参与度、组内影响力、团队合作力、协调能力等方面）。第二幕课上情景剧表演指导者得分记为整组作业成绩。

案例简介

本案例学习龋病预防相关内容，设计分为两幕进行。

第一幕主要学习不同的龋病预防方法，牙菌斑控制方法，氟化物防龋机制及窝沟封闭的适应证、操作步骤、注意事项。

第二幕主要学习氟化物的全身及局部应用方法、剂量、优缺点，预防性树脂充填的适应证、操作步骤，非创伤性修复治疗的适应证、操作步骤。通过提供临床案例及操作照片，希望学生学习并掌握龋病预防的方法、适应证、优缺点及操作步骤，熟悉龋病病因。通过文献的阅读，掌握口腔专业英语词汇。

关键词

氟化物，窝沟封闭，预防性树脂充填，非创伤性修复治疗

第一幕

　　李医生下乡支援山区口腔卫生建设，在当地进行口腔卫生宣教及治疗。某日，一位妈妈带着12岁的女儿前来就诊。

　　妈妈："李医生，你好！昨天隔壁邻居跟我说他家小孩在你这看牙了，给预防了虫牙，可以帮我闺女看看吗？"

　　李医生："好，那小朋友坐下来，让阿姨看看。小朋友有觉得牙齿哪里不舒服吗？"

　　小姑娘坐到简易牙椅上，摇摇头说没有。李医生为小姑娘做了仔细的检查，发现小姑娘前牙状况尚可，后牙可见少量软垢。46见𬌗面小龋洞，质软，探诊无明显酸痛，冷测同对照牙。其余磨牙窝沟深，未见明显龋坏，其中36颊侧见散在白斑，探诊略粗糙。

　　李医生："她已经有一颗虫牙了，以后还是要更加注意口腔卫生才行。"

　　妈妈马上对女儿说："听见了吗？每天让你刷牙，你都不好好刷，我还在刘婶那特意给你买了很贵的牙膏，你都给我浪费了。"接着又着急地转向李医生："你说她那么小，牙就长虫子，是不是平时吃得不好，营养跟不上，抵抗力弱啊？"

　　李医生："虫牙是一种通俗的叫法，我们专业上称为龋齿，也不是咱们想象的牙齿里面有虫子，它是一种很小的，小到肉眼看不见的细菌在慢慢侵蚀我们的牙齿，主要还是要靠刷牙把这些细菌刷掉，当然也有一些其他的预防方法。"

　　妈妈："那她这口牙齿还能预防吗？"

　　李医生："可以。已经坏了的那一颗，我们下次治疗，其他还没有坏的可以先做预防，预防虫牙发生。我先帮她把牙齿处理一下，一会儿再教你们平时怎么清洁牙齿。"

　　李医生选择先进行无痛的预防操作，这样可以让小姑娘减少第一次看牙的紧张。

　　李医生："我们先给后面还没有坏的大牙做窝沟封闭，降低以后发生虫牙的风险。然后给全口的牙齿涂一层保护漆，2～4小时后再进饮进食。这个保护漆呢，建议最好半年涂1～2次。"

　　李医生仔细地进行了标准的窝沟封闭操作，检查窝沟封闭完好后进行了全口涂氟。最后向母女二人介绍了一些保持口腔清洁的方法，让她们回去感受一下，并约明天再来治疗46。

患者资料	拟实施治疗计划
推断／假设	拟学习的问题

Act I

Dr. Li went to support oral health construction in rural areas, and carried out oral health education and treatment locally. One day, a mother came to the doctor's office with her 12-year-old daughter.

"Hello, Dr. Li. Yesterday, my neighbor told me that his child had a dental check with you to prevent caries. Can you have a look at my daughter's teeth?" the mother said.

"OK! Sit down, please. Let me have a look. Do you have any problems with your teeth?" Dr. Li asked.

The little girl sat down on the dental chair and shook her head. Dr. Li examined the girl's teeth carefully and found that the girl's anterior teeth were in good condition, while a small amount of soft dirt was visible on the posterior teeth. There were small carious cavities on the occlusal surface of 46, soft, no obvious pain on exploration, and the cold test was the same as that of the control tooth. The rest of the molars had deep pits and fissures without obvious caries. Scattered white spots were seen on 36 buccal surface, which was slightly rough when exploration probing.

"She already has a decayed tooth, and more attention should be paid to her oral health later." Dr. Li said.

The mother immediately said to her daughter, "Did you hear that? I told you to brush your teeth thoroughly, but you didn't. I also bought an expensive toothpaste from Aunt Liu for you, but you wasted it." Then she turned to Dr. Li anxiously, "Why does she have a worm tooth at such a young age? Is it because she doesn't eat well and the lack of nutrition decreases her resistance?"

"Worm tooth is a popular term, which is professionally known as dental caries. There is no worm in the tooth as we imagine while it is some little small bacteria, too small to be invisible, that eroded our teeth slowly. Whether they can be got rid of mainly depends on brushing teeth. Of course, there are also some other prevention methods." Dr. Li answered.

"Can her teeth still be prevented?" the mother asked.

"Yes. The decayed one can be treated, and the others can be prevented from cavities developing. I'll treat her un-decayed teeth first, and then tell you how to clean them correctly." Dr. Li answered.

Dr. Li first chose a less painful method of prevention, which could make the girl less nervous for about first dental visit.

"I will first perform the cavity sealing on teeth which have not been damaged to reduce the risk of getting decayed in the future. After that, I will apply protective paint to all her teeth. Don't let her eat or drink in 2–4 hours and don't brush her teeth tonight. It is recommended to apply this protective paint every six months." Dr. Li said.

Dr. Li performed a standard cavity sealing procedure carefully. After making sure that the cavity sealing had no obvious defects, fluoride was applied to the tooth surface. Finally, Dr. Li introduced some ways to keep oral hygiene to the mother and her daughter, and asked them to try ways out at home and come back to treat 46 tomorrow.

Patient information	Actions to take
Inference/Assumption	Question to study

第二幕

第二天，这位妈妈再次带女儿来到李医生的卫生室。

妈妈："李医生，我们来了。你昨天给她涂的保护漆是什么啊？半年涂1~2次，以后你走了，我们去哪里涂？可以自己买了回家涂吗？还能推荐给亲戚朋友。"

李医生："我走了没关系，卫生院就可以涂的，别担心。这个保护漆的使用还是需要一定的专业性指导，也不是对所有人都适用的，要医生判断和操作才行。"

妈妈："好吧，那我以后每半年带她来1次。"

李医生请小姑娘坐在牙椅上，为她处理了46（操作过程如图5所示）。治疗完成后嘱咐她们半年至少检查1次口腔，如出现问题及时处理。

卫生室的陈医生针对这两天的操作向李医生咨询了一些注意事项，并询问了李医生所在医院在龋病预防方面有没有更先进的方法。李医生向其介绍了预防性树脂充填和渗透树脂治疗，并简单介绍了目前尚在研究的一些预防方法。

陈医生："看来我还要多向乡亲们进行口腔卫生的宣教，做好基层预防工作。希望国内经济更快发展，进一步改善这里的医疗条件，让乡亲们都能拥有一口好牙。"

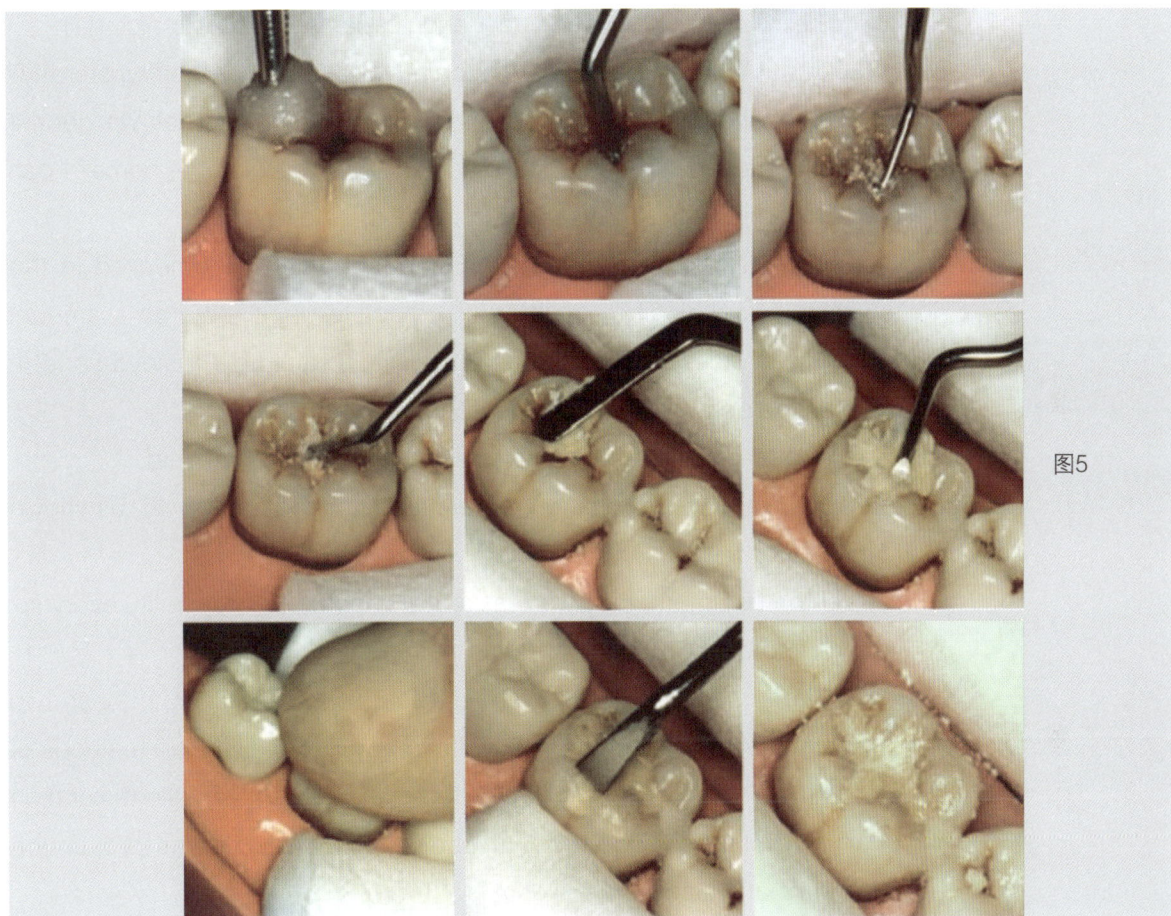

图5

患者资料	拟实施治疗计划
推断 / 假设	拟学习的问题

Act II

The next day, the mother and her daughter came to Dr. Li's clinic again.

"Hi Dr. Li! What is that protective paint you put on her teeth yesterday? You said it should be applied every six months. Where shall we get the treatment after you leave? Can I buy it myself and paint it at home? I can recommend it to my relatives and friends." the mother said.

"It doesn't matter. Don't worry because it can be smeared in the township hospital. The use of this protective paint requires a amount of certain professional guidance, and it is not suitable for everyone. It requires the doctor's judgment and operation." Dr. Li said.

"OK, I'll take her to revisit every six months." the mother said.

Dr. Li asked the girl to sit on the dental chair and treated 46, as shown in the Figure 5.

After the treatment, they were asked to check their oral cavity every six months and deal with oral problems in time.

Dr. Chen in the clinic asked Dr. Li about the precautions in these two days and asked whether his hospital had any more advanced methods of preventing dental caries. Dr. Li introduced the preventive resin restoration and resin infiltration therapy, and briefly introduced some prevention methods that are still under study.

"It seems that I have to do more oral health education to the villagers and do my best to grassroots prevention work. I hope our country's economy will develop rapidly so that we can improve medical conditions as soon as possible and all villagers can have a good oral condition." Dr. Chen said.

Patient information	Actions to take
Inference/Assumption	Question to study

编者：王一舟　江千舟

译者：陈荣丰

第四节　满嘴烂牙的小花

教学目标

掌握

1. 刷牙的方法及注意事项。

2. 牙线的使用方法。

3. 牙膏的基本作用。

熟悉

1. 口腔宣教的方法。

2. 漱口的方法。

3. 控制牙间隙菌斑的方法。

4. 漱口水的作用。

5. 牙刷的选择原则。

6. 常用的自我口腔保健方法。

了解

1. 功效牙膏的作用与特点。

2. 牙刷的设计和基本特点。

能力目标

通过预习、查阅文献，学习自我口腔保健用品及其使用方法，然后小组合作分析出案例中患者家长错误的口腔保健方法，并模拟椅旁宣教，教会患者正确的自我口腔保健方法。培养学生的临床素养和团队合作能力。

课程思政

口腔医疗机构向大众普及正确的自我口腔保健的相关知识，使其逐渐养成良好的口腔保健习惯，定期进行口腔检查，早发现、早诊断、早治疗，防微杜渐、长期坚持，量变引起质变，提升整体口腔健康水平。同时倡导家属对特殊人群给予口腔基本情况的关怀，比如低龄儿童、残疾人、老年人等。

课程设计

1. 课前学生10～12人为1组,课前2周发布案例,用于预习、查阅文献、分析案例。课上共6学时,其中第一幕讨论2学时(问题列举、提取学习目标15分钟,以问题为导向的讨论及解决第一幕的问题50分钟,总结反馈15分钟)。第二幕讨论4学时(问题列举、提取学习目标25分钟,以问题为导向的讨论及解决第二幕的问题70分钟,模拟椅旁宣教40分钟,总结反馈25分钟)。第一幕希望学生从回顾口腔接诊开始讨论,教师引导学生回顾口腔检查、龋病等相关内容,然后逐渐引出第一幕涉及的知识点:控制牙间隙菌斑的方法、X线片的重要性,为第二幕讨论做准备。第二幕希望学生从分析患者家长错误的口腔保健方法开始讨论,逐渐引出本幕的重点内容:刷牙的方法及注意事项、牙线的使用方法、牙膏的基本作用等。

2. 课后作业:第一次课程结束后的作业为预习并准备第二幕讨论,并将10～12人分为4小组,模拟针对特定人群进行口腔宣教的准备。第二次课程结束后的作业为1周内每人提交1篇关于自我口腔保健的科普论文。

3. 评价方式:课上表现占70%,作业占30%。课上表现使用自评、组内及组间互评、教师评价表评分(教师评价包括纪律性、参与度、组内影响力、团队合作力、协调能力等方面)。

案例简介

一位7岁的小女孩在学校口腔检查时发现有多颗牙龋坏。在医院经医生检查后发现患者患牙多、口腔卫生差,而且家长缺乏口腔保健知识。本案例设计分为两幕进行。

第一幕是讲述临床常见的一个接诊过程及患者家长对X线的误解。希望学生掌握如何向家长解释拍X线片的必要性和重要性,以及牙间隙菌斑的控制方法,同时复习口腔的基本检查方法。

第二幕是本章的重点,主要通过教师引导,学生找出家长错误的口腔保健观念,进而掌握正确的刷牙方法及注意事项、牙线的使用方法、牙膏的基本作用等,同时教会学生如何在临床上做好口腔卫生宣教,掌握与患者的沟通技巧,并熟悉自我口腔保健的其他方法。

通过此案例学习,引导学生掌握自我口腔保健的相关内容,并能熟练地应用于临床。

关键词

自我口腔保健,刷牙,牙刷,漱口水,牙线,牙膏

第一幕

　　1周前，在学校口腔检查中发现很多小学生都有不同程度的龋齿，7周岁的小花也不例外，检查结果显示有多颗龋齿。于是小花的爸爸王先生抽空带小花到口腔医院儿童口腔科就诊。

　　王先生："您好，想让医生给我女儿看一下牙齿，这是我的挂号纸和病历本。"

　　导诊："好的，请您稍等一下。（分诊）请您带着小朋友到1号诊室赵医生处就诊。"

　　赵医生看着一位穿戴整齐的男士带着一位穿着校服并且校服上有散在墨迹的小朋友走向自己。

　　王先生："请问您是赵医生吗？"

　　赵医生："是的，我是赵医生。请问有什么可以帮到您？"

　　王先生："赵医生您好，我女儿小花前几天在学校做口腔检查，发现她有一些蛀牙，我想让您再仔细检查一下。"

　　赵医生："好的，您家小朋友几岁了？"

　　王先生："7周岁。"

　　赵医生："小朋友的牙齿有没有不舒服？有没有痛过？"

　　王先生："我女儿以前都没说过牙齿不舒服，也没说过痛，所以她以前没看过牙医，这次学校检查，才知道她有蛀牙。"

　　赵医生："哦，那我们就先进行口腔检查。小朋友，坐在这个椅子上，你不用害怕，阿姨只是用小镜子照照你的牙齿，看牙齿上有没有虫子的城堡。"小花很乖地坐在牙椅上，并很配合赵医生的检查。

　　赵医生："小花爸爸，我刚才检查发现小花有8颗乳牙患龋，而且都比较严重，口腔卫生不是很好，有大量食物残渣还存留在牙齿表面和牙缝。因为龋坏比较严重，建议您先带小花去拍一个全口牙齿的X线片。"

　　王先生："啊？还要拍片啊，拍片有辐射，孩子这么小，我怕拍片影响她的发育，能不能不拍啊？反正她现在的牙齿以后都会换的，如果不影响她吃饭，我觉得治不治都无所谓的。"

　　经过赵医生再三解释，王先生最终还是带女儿拍摄了X线片。拍完X线片后，赵医生发现小花有8颗乳磨牙的牙冠部都有不同程度的低密度影像，其中1颗乳磨牙的牙冠部低密度影像已经到达髓腔，还有1颗乳磨牙的牙根下方有大面积低密度影像，已经将其下方的继承恒牙牙胚的骨硬板严重破坏。赵医生将相关情况向王先生进行了解释，王先生听了赵医生的解释后，深刻意识到小花牙齿龋坏的严重程度和拍片的必要性。

患者资料	拟实施治疗计划
推断 / 假设	拟学习的问题

Act I

A week ago, the school's oral examination found that many primary school students had different degrees of dental caries, and the 7-year-old Xiaohua was no exception. The examination results showed that there were many dental caries. So Mr. Wang, Xiaohua's father, took Xiaohua to the Children's Stomatology Department of Stomatological Hospital.

"Hello, I made an appointment with Dr. Zhao for my daughter. Here are my registration paper and medical record book." Mr. Wang said.

"OK, please wait a moment." the guide said.

"Please take your child to Dr. Zhao's office in clinic No.1." the triage said.

Dr. Zhao saw a well-dressed man and a child in a school uniform with scattered ink on it walking towards him.

"Excuse me, are you Dr. Zhao?" Mr. Wang asked.

"Yes, I am. What can I do for you?" Dr. Zhao said.

"Hello, Dr. Zhao. My daughter had an oral examination at school a few days ago, and found that she had some teeth decay. Could you please check it carefully again?" Mr. Wang said.

"OK, how old is your child?" Dr. Zhao asked.

"Seven years old." Mr. Wang answered.

"Are your child's teeth uncomfortable? Have they ever hurt?" Dr. Zhao asked.

"Xiaohua has never said that her teeth were uncomfortable or painful before, so she has never visited a dentist before. Only after this school examination did she know that she had tooth decay." Mr. Wang answered.

"Oh, let's have an oral examination first. Girl, sit on this chair. Don't be afraid. I just look at your teeth with a small mirror to see if there are castles of bugs on your teeth." Dr. Zhao said. Xiaohua sat on the dental chair quietly and cooperated with Dr. Zhao's examination.

"Mr. Wang, I just found that Xiaohua has eight deciduous teeth suffering from caries, and all of them are severe. The oral hygiene is not good, and a large amount of food residues still remain on the tooth surface and between the teeth. Because deciduous teeth caries is severe, it is recommended that Xiaohua should take a dental X-ray of her full teeth first." Dr. Zhao said.

"Huh? Does she have to take an X-ray? There is radiation when taking an X-ray. Xiaohua is so young and I am afraid that taking an X-ray will have a bad effect on her. Must she take an X-ray? Anyway, her teeth will be replaced. If it doesn't affect her eating, I think it doesn't matter whether she is cured or not." Mr. Wang said.

After repeated explanations by Dr. Zhao, Mr. Wang finally agreed to let Xiaohua take an X-ray. After Xiaohua took the X-ray, Dr. Zhao found that Xiaohua had 8 primary molars with varying degrees of radiolucent images on the crowns. Among them, the radiolucent images of the crowns of one primary molar had reached the pulp cavity, and there was a large area of radiolucent images under the root of one primary molar, which had seriously damaged the bone hard plate inheriting the permanent tooth germ below it. Dr. Zhao explained the relevant situation to Mr. Wang. After listening to Dr. Zhao's explanation, Mr. Wang was aware of the severity of Xiaohua's teeth and the necessity of taking the X-ray.

Patient information	Actions to take
Inference/Assumption	Question to study

第二幕

王先生："我女儿平时都不怎么吃糖，每天早上都会刷牙，用的牙膏都是进口的含氟牙膏，而且每天晚上也都会用儿童专用漱口水给她漱口，况且，小花以前在学校做过窝沟封闭，怎么还这么多蛀牙呢？是不是牙刷的毛太软了刷不干净？要不要换个电动牙刷？平时我们刷牙应该注意哪些方面呢？"

赵医生说："您可能还有很多地方没有做到位，其实口腔预防保健包括很多内容的，比如正确的刷牙、使用牙线、定期口腔检查等。至于刷牙需要注意哪些方面，一会儿我教您刷牙时会跟您讲的。"

王先生听完赵医生的解释后不禁感叹："口腔保健原来有这么多内容，自己还有很多功夫没做足。"于是请赵医生演示如何更好地进行自我口腔保健。赵医生就对小花和王先生进行了椅旁宣教。

患者资料	拟实施治疗计划
推断 / 假设	拟学习的问题

Act II

"Xiaohua doesn't eat much sugar usually. She brushes her teeth every morning. The toothpaste she uses is imported fluoride toothpaste and she rinses her mouth with children's mouthwash every night. Besides, Xiaohua had done cavity sealing at school before. Why are there still so many caries? Is the hair of the toothbrush too soft to brush cleanly? Should we change to an electric toothbrush? What should we pay attention to when brushing our teeth?" Mr. Wang asked.

"You may still have a lot to do. In fact, oral preventive health care includes a lot of content. For example, brushing your teeth correctly, flossing, regular oral examinations, etc. As for what you should pay attention to when brushing your teeth, I will tell you later." Dr. Zhao said.

After listening to Dr. Zhao's statement, Mr. Wang couldn't help but sigh. There was so much oral health care, and he still had a lot of effort to do, so he asked Dr. Zhao to demonstrate how to carry out self oral health care better. Dr. Zhao gave a chair-side education to Xiaohua and Mr. Wang.

Patient information	Actions to take
Inference/Assumption	Question to study

编者：曾素娟　李益玲

译者：刘珍妮　陈　彦

第二章
牙髓病和根尖周病

第一节　牙痛不是病，痛起来真"要命"

教学目标

掌握

1. 牙髓病病史采集的内容和问诊方法。

2. 牙髓的形态学特点。

3. 各型牙髓病的临床诊断方法、临床表现、诊断要点。

4. 牙髓炎的诊断程序和鉴别诊断思路。

熟悉

1. 牙髓的各种病理变化和分类。

2. 牙髓的功能及牙髓感觉神经纤维的特点。

了解

牙痛的鉴别诊断思路和所需鉴别的疾病。

能力目标

1. 通过本案例学习，学生能够评估患者状态，分析治疗的可行性。讨论如何更有效地使患者了解病情、接受治疗方案。

2. 牙髓病相关的致病菌及牙髓再生是近年牙体牙髓病学领域的研究热点。通过这一课程让学生学习如何发现问题、思考问题、查阅资料、提出新问题、设计实验方案等科研思路。

课程思政

1. 强调牙源性疾病的宣教以及社区、医院的防治措施的重要性。

2. 帮助学生快速进入医生角色，学会与患者沟通，关爱患者，更好地处理医患关系。引导学生在求解问题过程中能换位思考，重视患者的尊严和需求。

课程设计

1. 课前学生6～8人为1组分配任务，提出问题，列出教学目标中的重点与难点，查找资料。本案例以冷热痛为主要症状，讨论由龋病发展为牙髓炎的发病机制及临床特点，各型牙髓炎的诊断、鉴别诊断、治疗原则为主要学习目标。重点内容讨论时间约占80%，熟悉及了解的内容讨论时间约占20%。课堂采用随机选人答题、头脑风暴、抢答题的形式，提高学生的学习积极性及课堂参与度。

2. 课后作业：讨论结束后每人需交1篇牙髓炎的思维导图。

3. 评价方式：完成自评及互评表。评价讨论小组的整体水平及其他队员的参与度，比如参与讨论的积极性、聆听态度、沟通协调、课前准备、表达能力等。学生课堂表现、课后作业成绩作为平时成绩的一部分。

案例简介

本案例的设计分为两幕进行。

第一幕通过分析患者小蔡左下后牙疾病发展的过程探讨牙髓病的发病机制和临床特点，慢性牙髓炎的诊断、分型、鉴别诊断；希望学生学习并掌握由龋病发展为牙髓病的发病机制及临床特点；同时提供相关参考文献，帮助学生理解牙髓病病因及发病机制。

第二幕通过对小蔡左下后牙疾病变化的观测，分析急性牙髓炎的诊断、分型、鉴别诊断、影像学特点等以及根管治疗的原理、治疗原则、适应证与非适应证。希望学生学习急性牙髓病的发病机制和临床特点，掌握急性牙髓病的鉴别要点及鉴别诊断；提供相关参考文献，指导学生对急性牙髓病发病机制的理解，以及急性牙髓炎的临床处理原则。

关键词

急性牙髓炎，慢性牙髓炎，自发痛，阵发痛，冷热刺激疼痛，夜间痛

PBL Cases of Cariology and Endodontics (Student Edition)

第一幕

　　一天下午2：30，20岁的小伙子小蔡来到牙体牙髓科，说他左边下面从前往后数第四颗牙齿痛了2周，用冷水刷牙或吃烫的东西都会有明显疼痛，刚开始每次疼痛持续2～3分钟，这几天要持续十几分钟甚至半个小时；这颗牙齿1个月前在某诊所补过，在补牙之前也出现过疼痛。吃冷的东西就会痛那么几秒钟，只有当食物卡进洞里才会痛得厉害。补完之后好了一点儿，这才过了半个月，又开始痛了！孙医生问小蔡牙痛会不会影响睡眠，小蔡说晚上没有痛过。

　　孙医生为小蔡进行了口腔检查：口腔卫生良好。34远中𬌗面见复合树脂充填物。冷测敏感疼痛，冷刺激去除后疼痛持续一段时间，叩诊（－），无松动，其余牙未见明显异常。辅助检查（X线）如图6所示。

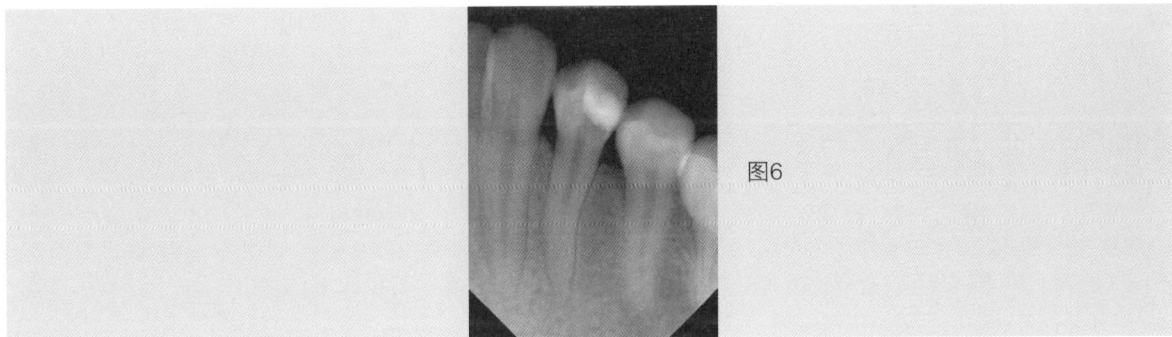

图6

　　孙医生问小蔡平时保持口腔卫生的习惯，小蔡说平常不怎么注意刷牙，连早晚各1次的刷牙也不能保证，牙缝经常塞东西，不痛也就不怎么在意。孙医生告诉小蔡患牙需要做的治疗。小蔡很惊讶，补牙这么复杂吗？还这么贵！小蔡要求回家考虑。

患者资料	拟实施治疗计划
推断 / 假设	拟学习的问题

Act I

A 20-year-old young man named Xiao Cai arrived at the Department of Endodontics at 2: 30 one afternoon. He said his fourth tooth on the lower left side, counting from front to back, had been painful for two weeks. It would cause obvious pain when brushing his teeth with cold water or eating hot food. In the beginning, the pain lasted for two or three minutes each time, but it would take more than ten minutes or even half an hour to stop the pain these days. The tooth was filled in the clinic a month ago, but before the tooth was filled, it also caused pain. Eating cold food would hurt for a few seconds, and only when the food was stuck in the cavity, would the pain be severe. After the tooth was filled, the symptoms eased a little. Half a month later, it began to hurt again! Dr. Sun asked Xiao Cai if the toothache would affect his sleep, and Xiao Cai said it caused no pain at night.

Dr. Sun performed an oral examination on Xiao Cai: his oral hygiene was good. Composite resin filling was found on the distal of 34 occlusion. The cold test showed sensitivity to pain. After the removal of the cold stimulus, the pain lasted for a while. No percussion pain, no tooth mobility, and no obvious abnormalities were observed in other teeth. Auxiliary examination (X-ray) was shown in the Figure 6:

Dr. Sun asked Xiao Cai about his usual oral hygiene habits. Xiao Cai said that he did not pay much attention to brushing his teeth, and could not even guarantee to brush his teeth twice in the morning and at night. Food was often impacted between the teeth. He didn't care if it didn't hurt. Dr. Sun told Xiao Cai that treatment was needed for his tooth. Xiao Cai was very surprised that the treatment was so complicated and expensive to fill a tooth. He had to consider it and went home.

Patient information	Actions to take
Inference/Assumption	Question to study

第二幕

3天后患者小蔡再次来到孙医生诊室。面容痛苦，精神状态欠佳。诉患牙从昨天下午开始剧烈疼痛，痛得昨晚都睡不着觉，吃了消炎药和止痛药都没有效。昨天开始痛的时候整个左边面部甚至连头都是痛的，现在感觉上下牙都痛，一直含着凉水才能舒服一点。

孙医生为小蔡进行了检查：血压108/76mmHg；34远中𬌗面见复合树脂充填物。冷测无不适，热诊疼痛，叩诊（±），无松动，其余牙未见明显异常。

孙医生向小蔡交代病情，告知治疗流程及费用并询问小蔡有无系统性疾病及药物过敏等，未发现相关病史。

小蔡签署知情同意书之后，孙医生对患牙34进行了治疗，并预约了下次治疗的时间。

患者资料	拟实施治疗计划
推断 / 假设	拟学习的问题

Act II

Three days later, Xiao Cai came to Dr. Sun's clinic again. His mental state was poor with a sad face. He complained that the tooth had been in severe pain since yesterday afternoon. The pain was so severe that he couldn't sleep last night. He took anti-inflammatory drugs and painkillers, but they didn't work. When the pain started yesterday, the whole left face and even the head were painful. Now he felt pain in both the upper and lower teeth. Only by holding cold water could he feel a bit more comfortable.

Dr. Sun examined Xiao Cai: his blood pressure was 108/76 mmHg; composite resin filling was found in the distal of 34 occlusion. The cold test showed no discomfort, the thermal test caused pain, percussion pain (±), no tooth mobility, and other teeth showed no obvious abnormalities.

Dr. Sun confessed his pathogenetic conditions to Xiao Cai, told him the treatment process and the cost, and asked whether Xiao Cai had any systemic diseases or drug allergies. No relevant medical history was found.

After Xiao Cai signed the informed consent form, Dr. Sun treated him patient and made an appointment for the subsequent treatment.

Patient information	Actions to take
Inference/Assumption	Question to study

编者：赵　健

译者：陈荣丰

第二节　牙神经的消亡史

教学目标

掌握

1. 各型根尖周炎的临床表现、诊断。

2. 急性根尖周炎的临床分期、排脓通道和排脓方式。

3. 急性根尖周脓肿与急性牙周脓肿的鉴别。

4. 根管治疗术的概念、病例选择和操作原则。

5. 根管充填材料的种类和性能。

6. 预防根管治疗并发症发生的方法。

7. 根管治疗后牙齿的变化特点，牙体修复的重要性及时机。

熟悉

1. 慢性根尖周炎的分型和病理变化。

2. 根管治疗术的原理和疗效评价标准。

3. 根管治疗并发症的种类及其发生的原因。

4. 根管治疗后牙体修复的材料与方法。

了解

1. 根尖周囊肿的形成理论。

2. 根管治疗术的发展概况。

3. 根管治疗并发症临床处理对策，避免不良预后。

4. 根管治疗后牙体修复的技术要点。

能力目标

通过本案例学习，学生要掌握根尖周病病史采集、口腔检查的一般方法，并正确书写病历。根据病史和临床检查对各型根尖周病做出诊断，并进行分期。分析根管充填材料的特点，启发、鼓励学生进行科研，优化材料性能。通过查阅文献增强对根管治疗及牙体修复的深刻认识。

课程思政

1. 加强科普宣教，使大众意识到牙痛不能单纯靠药物来治疗，增强大众对根尖周病及根管治疗的认识。

2. 熟悉临床病情告知技巧与注意事项。

3. 加强口腔诊疗中的人文关怀，探讨有哪些技巧和措施可减轻患者就诊时的恐惧。

4. 启发学生的爱国情怀，鼓励学生进行科学研究，探讨如何提高根充材料的封闭性、生物相容性，促进根充材料的国产化。

PBL Cases of Cariology and Endodontics (Student Edition)

课程设计

1. 课前2周发布案例，课前学生以8～10人1组进行自主学习，阅读分析案例后提出问题，以问题为导向进行文献阅读，搜集资料。课前自主学习4学时，课上案例讨论2学时（其中脑力激荡10分钟、列举问题5分钟、讨论及引导55分钟、总结10分钟）。希望学生由"咬物痛"开始，逐步讨论出根尖周炎的分类、临床表现、诊断和鉴别诊断，以及疾病之间的发展与转归。

2. 课后作业：复习前面学习过的龋病、非龋性疾病、牙髓病的相关内容，制作1份有关"牙痛"的鉴别诊断的思维导图，需每人独立完成1份。

3. 评价方式：课上表现占70%、作业占30%。课上表现使用自评、组内及组间互评、教师评价表评分（教师评价包括纪律性、参与度、组内影响力、团队合作力、协调能力等方面）。

关键词

咬物痛，窦道，根尖周炎，根管治疗，器械分离，牙体修复，微渗漏

案例简介

患者林先生，因左上后牙咬物痛就诊，医生检查后发现25牙冠远中邻𬌗面龋损达髓腔，探及根管口，无探痛，叩诊（+++），Ⅱ°松动，冷测无反应，未探及明显牙周袋。X线片示：25牙冠低密度影达髓腔，根尖区无明显低密度影。医生建议25行根管治疗，患者未做任何处理。3个月后患者再次因为同一颗牙就诊，医生检查后发现25远中邻𬌗面大面积龋坏，叩诊（±），无明显松动，颊侧根尖区牙龈可见窦道，按压有脓液溢出。X线片示：25牙冠低密度影达髓腔，根尖区大面积低密度影。医生耐心地向林先生详细解释了病情及治疗方案。最后林先生接受了医生的建议，进行了根管治疗。

本案例主要学习根尖周病相关内容，设计分为两幕进行。

第一幕主要学习根尖周炎的分类、临床表现、诊断和鉴别诊断，以及疾病之间的发展与转归。让学生对各型根尖周炎进行分类，同时提供参考文献，希望学生深刻理解各型根尖周炎的临床表现和诊断。

第二幕主要学习根管治疗术的定义、根管治疗的并发症及预防方法；根管治疗后牙体的变化特点、牙体修复的重要性与时机。通过参考文献和临床案例，让学生深刻理解根管治疗术的概念和操作原则，以及根管治疗后牙体修复的重要性。

第一幕

林先生，65岁，因左上后牙肿痛，就诊于口腔医院牙体牙髓科。

王医生见林先生表情非常痛苦，便问："您牙齿哪里不舒服？"

林先生："我牙痛啊，痛得受不了。"

王医生："哪个地方痛，从什么时候开始的？"

林先生："左边上面的牙痛，痛了3天了。"

王医生："遇到冷热水痛吗？"

林先生："现在遇到冷热水不痛，1个月前碰到冷热水就痛得厉害，有时候晚上痛得睡不着。后来不痛了，我以为好了，没想到现在又痛了，而且痛得受不了。"

王医生："您是怎么个痛法，阵痛还是持续痛？"

林先生："刚开始是有点胀胀的，用力咬牙就会觉得好一点，我也没在意。前天开始感觉疼痛加重了，而且咬牙时会更痛。"

王医生："是钝痛还是跳痛？"

林先生："前面两天我感觉都是钝痛，昨天开始都是一跳一跳地痛，昨晚痛得都没睡好，今天早上就赶紧过来了。我现在觉得这个牙好像长长了，嘴巴轻轻一合就能碰到这个牙，就会特别痛，医生，你赶紧给我看看是怎么回事？"

王医生："我现在给您检查，请您放松，不会很痛的，我会轻轻地，检查过程中如果您感觉到痛或其他不适，请举一下左手，我会立即停下来。为了您的安全考虑，请您不要随便举起右手或抓我的手。必要的话会拍X线片。"

王医生对林先生的口腔进行了检查。

临床检查：25牙冠远中邻𬌗面龋损达髓腔，探及根管口，探痛（−），叩诊（+++），Ⅱ°松动，冷测无反应，未探及明显牙周袋。

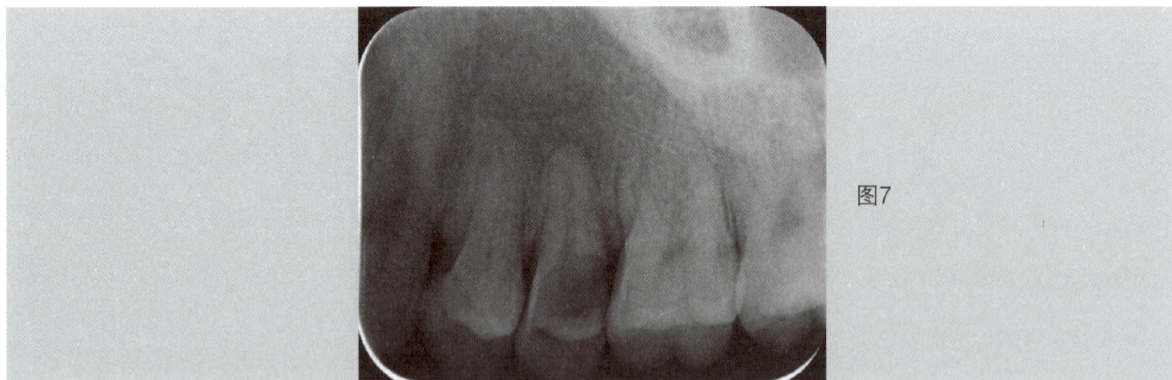

图7

X线片示：25冠部低密度影达髓腔，根尖区无明显低密度影（图7）。

医生向患者解释了病情，介绍了治疗方案和疗程，患者由于无时间复诊，要求择期治疗。

3个月后，林先生再次来到牙体牙髓科。

林先生："医生，上次从您这走了之后又痛了好几天，而且脸都肿了，后来到社区医院打了'消炎针'后慢慢地就不痛了。最近1个月牙龈上面长了个脓包，好了又长，反反复复，但是牙齿基本不痛了。牙齿都不痛了，不是应该好了吗，怎么还会长脓包啊？"

王医生："我需要给您做进一步的检查，需要拍X线片。"

临床检查：25远中邻𬌗面大面积龋坏，探及根管口，探痛（－），叩诊（±），冷测无反应，无明显松动。颊侧根尖区牙龈可见窦道，按压有脓液溢出。

王医生从脓包的地方插进一根牙胶尖，然后让患者拍X线片（图8）。

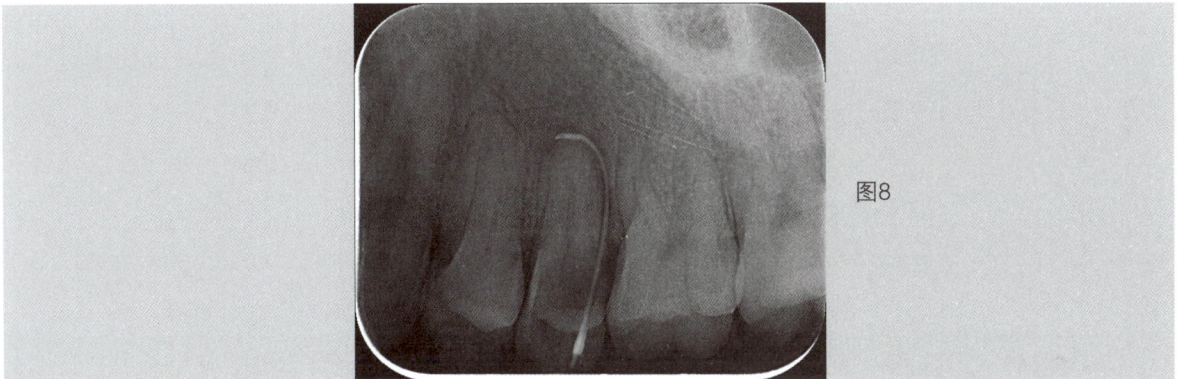

图8

X线片示：25根尖区大面积低密度影。示踪牙胶尖至25根尖区。

患者资料	拟实施治疗计划
推断 / 假设	拟学习的问题

Act I

Mr. Lin, 65 years old, visited the Department of Endodontics of the Stomatology Hospital with toothache and swollen gums in the left upper posterior area.

Seeing Mr. Lin with a harrowing expression, Dr. Wang asked, "What is wrong with your teeth?"

"I had a toothache, and the pain is unbearable." Mr. Lin answered.

"Which area hurts, and when did it start?" Dr. Wang asked.

"The left upper tooth which has been painful for 3 days." Mr. Lin answered.

"Does it hurt when you drink hot or cold water?" Dr. Wang asked.

"Now it doesn't hurt in hot or cold water, but a month ago it hurt so much when I drank hot or cold water that sometimes I couldn't sleep at night. Later, I didn't feel the pain, and I thought it was over, but now it hurts again, and the pain is unbearable." Mr. Lin said.

"What kind of pain do you have, a little or persistent pain?" Dr. Wang asked.

"At first, it was a little bloated and uncomfortable. When I bit down hard, I felt better. I did not care. The day before yesterday the pain started to get worse and was even more painful when biting." Mr. Lin answered.

"Is it dull pain or throbbing pain?" Dr. Wang asked.

"I've had a dull pain for the first two days, and it's been throbbing since yesterday. I couldn't sleep well last night because of the pain. Now I feel as if this tooth has grown longer, and my mouth can touch this tooth when I gently close it, which makes it extremely painful. Doctor, would you please tell me what is going on?" Mr. Lin said.

"I give you an examination now. Take it easy. It will not be very painful. During the examination, if you feel pain or other discomforts, please raise your left hand, and I will immediately stop. For your safety, please do not lift your right hand or grab my hand. If necessary, an X-ray will be taken." Dr. Wang said.

Dr. Wang examined Mr. Lin's mouth.

Clinical examination: the caries of the distal proximal and occlusal surface of the crown of 25 reached the pulp cavity; root canal opening was detected; probing pain (−); percussion pain (++); tooth mobility (II°); no response to cold test; no obvious periodontal pocket was detected.

X-ray showed: radiolucent shadow in the crown of 25 reached the pulp cavity; no obvious radiolucent shadow in the apical region (Figure 7).

The doctor explained the condition and described the treatment plan and courses of treatment. Mr. Lin asked for elective treatment due to a lack of time for follow-up.

Three months later, Mr. Lin came back to the Department of Endodontics.

"Doctor, I have been in pain for several days since I left your place last time, and my face was swollen. Then I went to the community hospital and got an anti-inflammatory injection the pain gradually disappeared. In the past month, an abscess grew on the gum, which has healed and grown over and over again, but the tooth is basically painless. So I think the tooth should be fine now since it doesn't hurt, why are there still pustules?" Mr. Lin said.

"I need to give you further examination and you need to take an X-ray." Dr. Wang said.

Clinical examination: 25 large caries on the distal proximal and occlusal surfaces; root canal opening was probed; probing pain (−); percussion pain (±); no response to cold test; no obvious tooth mobility; sinus tracts were visible in the gingiva of the buccal apical area, and pus overflowed by pressure.

Dr. Wang inserted a gutta-percha point from the abscess and then asked Mr. Lin to take an X-ray (Figure 8).

X-ray showed: a large radiolucent shadow in the apical area of 25 roots. Tracing the gutta-percha point to the 25 apical zones.

Patient information	Actions to take
Inference/Assumption	Question to study

第二幕

王医生经过检查，并对比了两次的X线片后回复到："您的牙齿现在有慢性根尖周炎，需要做根管治疗，做完后还需要做个牙冠将牙齿保护起来。"

林先生："根管治疗是什么意思啊？治疗过程是怎样的啊？治疗过程中需要吃药吗？需要来几次？"王医生耐心地对林先生解释了什么是根管治疗，并告知治疗过程中可能会出现疼痛、肿胀等情况。最后林先生接受了医生的建议进行根管治疗。

做完根管治疗后，林先生不太想做牙冠，说："医生，牙冠一定要做吗？过段时间再做行吗？不做行吗？"

患者资料	拟实施治疗计划
推断 / 假设	拟学习的问题

Act Ⅱ

Dr. Wang examined and compared the two X-ray films. "Your tooth suffers chronic apical periodontitis and needs root canal therapy, after which a crown will be made to protect it." replied Dr. Wang after examing and comparing the two X-ray films.

"What does root canal therapy mean? What is the approximate procedure? Do I need to take medicine during the treatment? How many visits are required?" Mr. Lin asked. Dr. Wang patiently explained to Mr. Lin what root canal therapy was, and informed him that there might be pain and swelling during the treatment. Finally, Mr. Lin accepted the doctor's recommendation to have root canal therapy.

After the root canal therapy, Mr. Lin did not want to do the crown, and said, "Doctor, do I have to do the crown? Can I do it later? Is it OK not to do it?"

Patient information	Actions to take
Inference/Assumption	Question to study

编者：张文娟

译者：温思怡

第三节　牙外伤引起的根尖周病

教学目标

掌握

1. 根管治疗术的概念及操作。

2. 根管再治疗的适应证及术前评估。

3. 根尖手术的适应证。

4. 根尖囊肿的临床及病理表现。

熟悉

1. 根管治疗疗效评价标准。

2. 根管外科手术的分类。

了解

1. 根管治疗的并发症及根管治疗后的疾病的病因。

2. 根尖手术的步骤和方法。

能力目标

1. 通过本案例中牙外伤的发生，逐渐转化为根尖周病的疾病发展过程，引导学生将牙外伤与根尖周病相关专业知识与该病例有机的结合，从而培养学生学习牙体牙髓病学专业知识的能力。

2. 本案例中的整个疾病发展过程是循序渐进的，从中可以启发学生以此病例为模板，建立一个以牙外伤或根尖周病的临床实验模型，进行相关临床科研知识的研究与学习。

3. 本案例中根尖周病发展到后期转变为难治性的根尖周病，治疗方案也选择了更加复杂的根尖手术，涉及比较多的课外知识，由此可引导学生主动查阅课外文献及相关资料，培养学生积极主动的自学能力。

课程思政

1. 本案例中的患者因牙外伤导致牙龈肿胀而就诊。在就诊过程中，医生的整个问诊过程都是以患者为中心的，设身处地为患者去着想，由此可启发学生对患者的人文关怀思想。

2. 本案例中，在患者的就诊过程中，医生仔细询问了患者牙龈肿胀的病史并做了完善的口腔检查，并且根据诊断做了正确的治疗计划，也详细告知了患者治疗的风险及预后等情况。医生的作风严谨，一丝不苟，从而可以培养学生高尚的品德、医德和政治素养。

课程设计

1. 课前学生以10～12人为1组，设置1名组长，1名记录员。以牙外伤的分类与临床表现、根尖周炎的病因与治疗原则、根管治疗、根管再治疗的方式、根管治疗后的疾病等为主要学习目标，分配任务，提出问题，以问题为导向方式列出学习重点，一起查找资料。课堂上小组组长引导学生自由讨论50分钟，记录员记录讨论的问题及内容，分析总结20分钟，教师点评总结10分钟。

2. 课后作业：讨论结束后1周内需上交1份本课程问题分析的PPT。

3. 评价方式：课上表现使用自评、组内及组间互评、教师评价表评分（教师评价包括纪律性、参与度、组内影响力、团队合作力、协调能力等方面）。

案例简介

本案例学习牙外伤、根尖周病、根尖手术等相关内容，设计分为两幕进行。第一幕主要表现牙外伤的病史与临床表现，希望学生学习并掌握牙外伤转归为根尖周病的病理发展过程，让学生认识到检查对于根尖周病诊断的重要性。提供辅助的影像学检查，重点让学生掌握根尖周病的治疗方法、根管治疗的步骤、根管再治疗的适应证，了解根管治疗后的疾病病因等。

第二幕进一步提供复诊后的口腔检查及影像学检查，希望学生讨论根尖周病复发的原因，同时让学生学习并掌握根尖囊肿的临床及病理表现。最后结合案例让学生讨论根管外科手术的种类，主要要求学生掌握根尖手术的适应证，了解根尖手术的步骤和方法。

关键词

牙外伤，咬合创伤，根管再治疗，显微根尖手术，慢性根尖周炎

第一幕

26岁的小陈来口腔医院看病，挂了杨医生的专家号，在诊室外候诊，护士在询问患者病情及病史后让其等待。10分钟后，小陈坐在了治疗椅上。

小陈："医生，这次来主要是因为我的左上前牙咬东西时会感到疼痛。"

杨医生："这种疼痛有多长时间了？"

小陈："大概有2个多月了。"

杨医生："左上前牙以前是做过什么治疗吗？"

小陈回答道："是的，左上前牙曾在10年前受到过外伤，打篮球的时候撞伤了，当时撞得挺痛的，出了一点血，但是我觉得没什么大碍就没去管它，没想到过了不久牙齿周围便出现了肿胀，我去社区的医院看过一次医生，当时医生好像是给我做了一个什么根管治疗吧。"

杨医生："那当时做完治疗后的情况呢？"

小陈："做完根管治疗后不久，症状便消退了，一直也没什么事，直到2个月前不慎咬到硬物后便开始疼痛，然后就一直持续到现在。"

杨医生听完小陈的陈述，仔细检查了小陈的口腔情况（图9）：21轻度变色，舌侧见牙色充填体，叩诊（+），Ⅰ°松动，冷测无反应，PD为10mm，BOP（+），唇侧牙龈颜色正常，根尖区未见明显窦道口，腭侧牙龈略肿胀，未扪及波动感。11轻度变色，近中切端缺损，叩诊（−），无松动，冷测同正常对照牙，牙龈未见明显肿胀。邻牙12、22未见明显异常。前牙Ⅱ°深覆𬌗，Ⅲ°深覆盖，后牙咬合关系正常。

杨医生说："你这次的症状可能是这颗做过治疗的牙齿引起的，所以我建议你先拍摄一个CT来确诊一下。"

小陈欣然答应后便去放射科行CBCT检查。

小陈很快便做完了影像学检查，回到了杨医生的诊室，杨医生仔细查看了小陈的影像学检查。

CBCT示：21根管内见高密度充填影像达根尖，充填影像稍稀疏，根尖区见低密度影像，唇腭侧骨板尚存（图9）。

　　杨医生告知小陈："你这次的症状主要是左上前牙引起的，我们需要对它重新行根管治疗，若再治疗失败可能还需行根尖手术。"小陈在医生和护士的解释中充分了解了自己的病情及费用后签署了知情同意书，杨医生开始对21行根管再治疗。

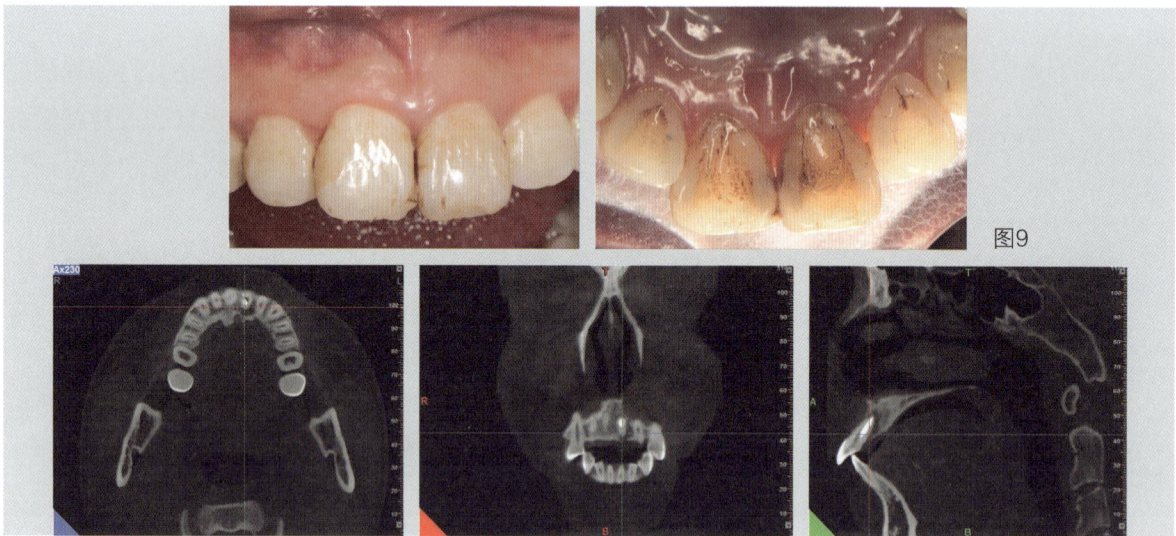

图9

患者资料	拟实施治疗计划
推断 / 假设	拟学习的问题

Act Ⅰ

Xiao Chen, 26 years old, came to the dental hospital to visit a dentist. While he was waiting outside the clinic, the nurse asked Xiao Chen about his condition and medical history and then told him to wait. Ten minutes later, Xiao Chen sat on Dr. Yang's dental chair.

"Doctor, the main reason for my visit is that my upper left front teeth would feel pain and discomfort when biting something." Xiao Chen said.

"How long have you been in this pain?" Dr. Yang asked.

"It's been more than two months." Xiao Chen answered.

"Have you had previous treatment on your upper left front tooth?" Dr. Yang asked.

Xiao Chen replied, "Yes, I had a trauma to my upper left front tooth 10 years ago. I was injured when I was playing basketball. It was quite painful and bled a little, but I didn't think it was serious so I left it alone. I didn't expect swelling and discomfort around the tooth soon after. I went to the community hospital to visit the doctor once. At that time, the doctor seemed to have done root canal treatment for me, I think."

"What about the situation after the treatment?" Dr. Yang asked.

"My symptoms subsided shortly after the root canal therapy, and it was fine until two months ago when I started to experience pain and discomfort after accidentally biting a hard object. Then it has continued until now." Xiao Chen said.

After listening to Xiao Chen's statement, Dr. Yang carefully examined Xiao Chen's oral cavity: 21 mild discolorations, lingual dental-colored filling body, percussion pain (+), tooth mobility (I°), no response to cold examination, PD=10mm, BOP (+), normal gingival color on the labial side, no obvious sinus opening in the apical area, slightly swollen gingiva on the palatal side, no sense of palpable volatility. 11 mild discolorations, proximal mesial incisal defect, percussion pain (−), no tooth mobility, cold test as normal teeth, no significant swelling of the gingiva. The adjacent 12 and 22 showed no significant abnormalities. The anterior deep overbite (II°) and deep overjet (III°), and the posterior teeth had normal occlusal relationships.

Dr. Yang told Xiao Chen, "Your symptoms this time may be caused by this tooth that has been treated, so I suggest you take a CBCT examination to confirm the diagnosis."

Xiao Chen readily agreed and then went to the radiology department for a CBCT examination.

Xiao Chen soon finished the imaging examination and returned to Dr. Yang's office, where Dr. Yang was carefully reviewing Xiao Chen's imaging examination results.

CBCT showed that radiopaque filling images up to the apex were seen in the root canal of 21, and the filling images were slightly sparse. Radiolucent images were found in the apical area, and the labial-palatal bone plate was still present (Figure 9).

Dr. Yang told Xiao Chen, "Your symptoms are mainly caused by the upper left anterior tooth. We need to perform root canal treatment again, and if the retreatment fails, endodontic surgery is required." Xiao Chen signed an informed consent form after the doctor and nurse explained his condition and the cost. Dr. Yang started to perform root canal retreatment on 21.

Patient information	Actions to take
Inference/Assumption	Question to study

第二幕

1年后，小陈回到了杨医生处复诊。小陈告知杨医生1年前左上前牙行根管再治疗后症状有所缓解，但近几日在无明显诱因下出现了牙龈肿胀。

杨医生在检查小陈口腔情况后发现：21腭侧牙龈见明显肿胀，有压痛，故行影像学检查。CBCT示：21根管内见高密度充填影像达根尖，根尖见大面积低密度影像，腭侧低密度影累及切牙管，腭侧骨板见破坏影像（图10）。

杨医生告知小陈21根管再治疗后效果不理想，需行根尖手术，在小陈的同意下杨医生对21行微创显微根尖手术＋腭侧囊肿刮除术，术后恢复情况良好。

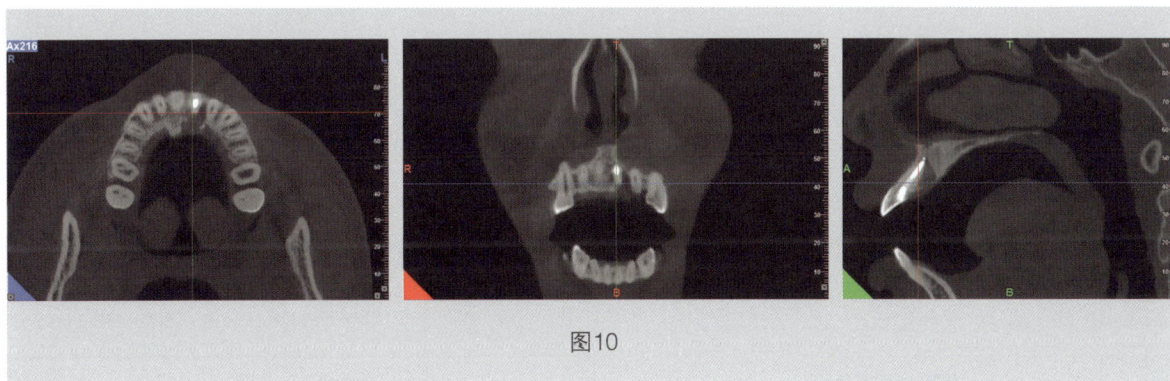

图10

患者资料	拟实施治疗计划
推断／假设	拟学习的问题

Act II

One year later, Xiao Chen returned to Dr. Yang for a follow-up visit. Xiao Chen informed Dr. Yang that his symptoms had subsided after root canal retreatment of his upper left front tooth a year ago, but in recent days he had experienced gingival swelling and discomfort without apparent cause.

After examining Xiao Chen's oral cavity, Dr. Yang found that the palatal gingiva of 21 was significantly swollen with pressure pain. Therefore, imaging examination was performed. CBCT showed that: 21 radiopaque filling images were seen in the root canal up to the root tip, large radiolucent images were seen in the apical area, radiolucent shadows on the palatal side involved the incisal canal, and destruction images were seen on the palatal bone plate (Figure 10).

Dr. Yang informed Xiao Chen that the results of 21 root canal retreatment were not satisfactory and that endodontic surgery was needed. Dr. Yang performed minimally invasive endodontic microsurgery+palatal periradicular curettage on 21 with Xiao Chen's consent. Xiao Chen recovered well after the surgery.

Patient information	Actions to take
Inference/Assumption	Question to study

编者：刘　晓

译者：温思怡

PBL Cases of Cariology and Endodontics (Student Edition)

第四节　一例牙周牙髓联合病变引发的思考

教学目标

掌握

1. 牙周牙髓联合病变的交通途径、相互影响。

2. 牙周牙髓联合病变的临床表现及治疗原则。

3. 牙周牙髓联合病变的诊断程序和鉴别诊断思路。

熟悉

1. 牙周脓肿和牙槽脓肿的诊断与鉴别诊断。

2. 牙周炎和牙髓炎的治疗。

3. 牙周牙髓联合病变的预后。

了解

1. 牙周牙髓联合病变的发病机制及病理变化。

2. 疾病治疗方案的综合设计。

能力目标

通过本案例学习，提高学生对牙周牙髓联合病变基本知识的理解能力，理论联系实际，为临床技能操作打好基础。通过学习牙周牙髓联合病变的交通途径、相互影响等相关研究，培养学生科研思维，鼓励学生进行科学研究。

课程思政

通过展示人文关怀及有效的医患沟通（如术前耐心细致的沟通，时刻观察患者的反应，安排护士陪同拍片，术后医嘱，预留科室电话等），培养学生要具有博爱的胸怀，用关怀和帮助的心态面对患者，学会用易于患者理解的语言与患者交流。

课程设计

1. 课前学生8～10人为1组，设置1名组长，1名记录员。阅读案例后提出问题，以问题为导向方式列出学习重点，由组长分配任务，查找相关资料。课前文献阅读4学时，课上案例讨论2学时（脑力激荡10分钟、问题列举5分钟、讨论55分钟、总结10分钟）。讨论的时间分配：掌握的内容：熟悉和了解的内容为4∶1。以牙髓源性牙周牙髓联合病变的病因、诊断、鉴别诊断等为学习目标。讨论引导方向：希望学生能由"牙龈脓包"开始讨论，涉及的知识点包括主诉牙病史的采集、牙周牙髓联合病变的解剖生理及分型、牙周牙髓联合病变的诊断依据及其鉴别诊断、诊疗过程中的人文关怀及有效的医患沟通。

2. 课后作业：讨论结束后每人需交1份本次课的PPT并完成课后作业。

3. 评价方式：及时完成自我评价及对他人的评价，提交一份自评表及组内互评表。

关键词

咬物痛，牙龈脓肿，牙周袋，
牙周牙髓联合病变

案例简介

覃某，女，62岁。左下后牙反复牙龈脓包3月余，近2周来咬物疼痛加重，自服3天消炎药，脓包仍未消退，就诊。医生检查发现36近中邻𬌗面大面积金属充填物，远中邻面探及深龋坏，冷测无反应，叩诊（＋＋），Ⅰ°松动。颊侧距离龈缘约5mm见一软性包块，波动感，刺破后溢脓，颊侧探及宽而深的牙周袋，探及根分叉，PD近10mm。检查全口状况后，经与患者沟通，建议拍摄X线片以辅助诊断。最后根据病史及相关辅助检查给患者做出治疗计划。

本案例的设计分为两幕进行。

第一幕主要引导学生进行病史的采集，牙周牙髓联合病变的解剖生理及分型，牙周牙髓联合病变的诊断依据、鉴别诊断，诊疗过程中的人文关怀及有效的医患沟通。希望学生学习并掌握牙周牙髓联合病变的诊断依据及鉴别诊断；提供相关参考文献，帮助教师指导学生对牙周牙髓联合病变的理解。

第二幕主要引导学生进行有效的医患沟通，给患者制订合理的治疗方案；提供临床案例的辅助检查X线片，重点让学生掌握综合治疗方案的制订及病历书写。

第一幕

　　早上8：00，牙体牙髓科王医生和护士开始一天的工作。"覃小英？请问覃小英在吗？"

　　接诊的王医生看到覃阿姨面色憔悴、愁容满面地走进诊室，以至于叫了两次名字才听到。刚一进来就迫不及待地说："医生啊，我的牙不知道怎么了，牙肉那里长了个包，原本只是有时候吃东西会不太舒服，但是前两天突然就痛得要命啊，感觉整个人都不好了，吃了好多消炎药都没用，这怎么回事啊，是不是得肿瘤了？"

　　王医生："阿姨，先请坐，不要着急，我们慢慢说。请问，这是您的病历吗？您叫什么名字？"病历上面显示家住广州，1958年出生，职业销售，本地医保。

　　护士引导患者坐在椅位上，患者紧张地点头回应"是我的病历，我叫覃小英"。

　　王医生询问患者有无高血压、心脏病、糖尿病，药物过敏史，均得到否定答复。患者告知最近睡眠质量不好。

　　王医生："您主要是哪里不舒服？"

　　覃阿姨："左边牙痛。"

　　王医生："您主要是感觉牙痛还是牙肉痛，能明确是上面痛还是下面痛吗？"

　　覃阿姨："牙肉那里鼓了个包，下面痛"，边说患者就用手指向牙齿。医生大概看到了35、36的位置有个脓包。

　　王医生："发现大约有多长时间了？之前有没有肿过？"

　　"这次大概有2周了吧，我不太记得了，唉！一直没理它，没想到就这样了。我倒是记得之前也有过一次，是3个月前的事了，但是没管它就好了。"

　　"那您的牙齿有治疗过吗？"

　　"没有，去药店买了药，吃了也没用"。说着从包里拿出剩下的消炎药，"医生，您看，就是这些。"

　　王医生示意患者躺下，张开口进行检查，并告知患者检查过程不用紧张，有问题举左手，检查过程中不要随意讲话以免医疗器械锋利扎伤口腔黏膜。护士见患者紧张，主动握住患者的手，不时安慰，并为她盖上小被子保暖。

王医生开始对患者进行视诊、探诊、叩诊等常规口腔检查，冷测前先测试26、25，再测试35、36，告知患者如有疼痛或其他不适举左手示意。轻拉患者口角，发现患者口唇较干，嘱咐护士涂抹护唇油，以免检查过程中引起患者的不适。检查过程中发现患者36近中邻𬌗面大面积金属充填物，远中邻面探及深龋坏，冷测无反应，叩诊（++），I°松动。颊侧距离龈缘约5mm见一软性包块，轻轻按压发现波动感，表面麻醉后刺破溢脓，颊侧探及宽而深的牙周袋，探及根分叉，PD近10mm。35、37牙体未见龋坏，叩诊（－），冷测同正常对照牙，无松动。46𬌗面见一牙色充填体，边缘有勾拉、粗糙感，叩诊（－），冷测同正常对照牙，无松动。16𬌗面大面积金属充填物，21近中见一牙色充填体，近中有食物嵌塞，叩诊（－），冷测无反应，无松动。38、48存，无对颌。全口口腔卫生一般，牙龈轻度红肿，探诊出血。检查后王医生告知覃阿姨大概情况，经沟通后建议患者拍摄X线片辅助诊断，患者表示配合。覃阿姨焦虑明显减轻，并告知医生，检查过程中未有任何不适，对医生护士表示信任。

接着王医生安排护士陪同覃阿姨去拍了X线片（图11）。

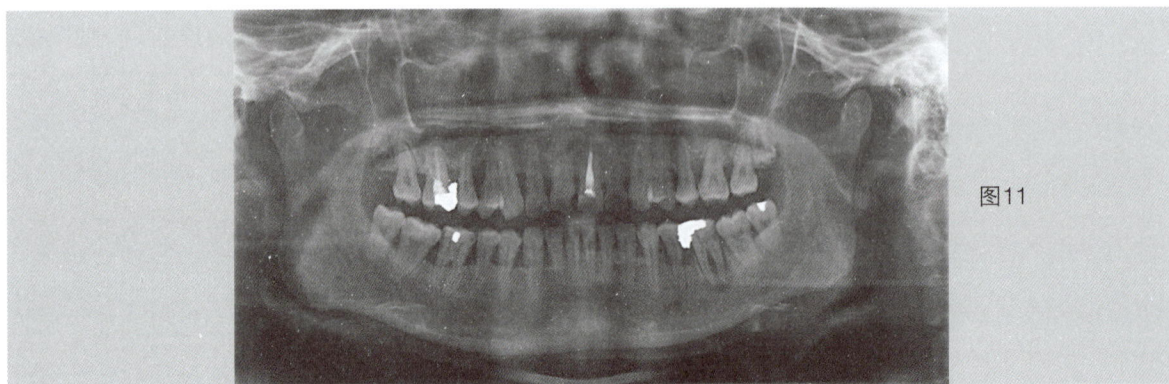

图11

患者资料	拟实施治疗计划
推断 / 假设	拟学习的问题

Act I

It's 8: 00 in the morning. Dr. Wang and the nurse from the Department of Endodontics began their work. "Xiaoying Qin? Is Xiaoying Qin here?"

Dr. Wang saw Ms. Qin walking into the office with a lean face. He called her name twice before she heard it. Ms. Qin came in and couldn't wait to say, "Doctor, I don't know what's wrong with my teeth. There is a bulge in the gum. It just makes me uncomfortable to eat sometimes, but the pain suddenly became so bad two days ago that I felt terrible. A lot of anti-inflammatories are useless, what's going on? Is there a tumor?"

"Please sit down first. Don't worry. Is this your medical record? What is your name?" Dr. Wang asked. The medical record showed that she lived in Guangzhou, was born in 1958, was a professional salesman, and had local medical insurance.

The nurse guided the patient to sit on the chair, and the patient nodded nervously in response, "This is my medical record. My name is Qin Xiaoying."

Dr. Wang asked whether the patient had high blood pressure, heart disease, diabetes, or any history of drug allergy, and received negative answers. Ms. Qin said that she hadn't been sleeping well lately.

"What's the main problem?" Dr. Wang asked.

"Left toothache." Ms. Qin answered.

"You mainly feel toothache or gingival pain? Can you tell whether it hurts in the upper or the lower site?" Dr. Wang asked.

"There's a bulge in the gums. Down there." Ms. Qin answered. She pointed to the tooth while saying that. The doctor probably saw a pustule in 35 and 36.

"How long has it been since it was discovered? Have you had any swelling before?" Dr. Wang asked.

"It has been about two weeks. I can't remember. I had been busy working and ignored it, and I didn't expect it to be like this. I remembered that it happened once before, about three months ago, but it was fine to leave it alone." Ms. Qin answered.

"Have you had your teeth treated?" Dr. Wang asked.

"No, I went to the pharmacy and bought some medicine, but it didn't help." Ms. Qin took the rest of the medicine out of her bag. "Here it is, Doctor."

Dr. Wang suggested the patient lie down and open her mouth for examination, and told the patient not to be nervous during the examination, to raise her left hand if there was any problem and not to speak during the examination to avoid sharp medical instruments puncturing the oral mucosa. Seeing that the patient was nervous, the nurse took the initiative to hold the patient's hand, comforted her from time to time, and took a small quilt for her to keep warm. Dr. Wang began routine oral examinations such as inspection, probing and percussion. Before the cold test, the patient was tested 26 and 25, and then tested 35 and 36. Dr. Wang told the patient to raise her left hand if she felt pain or discomfort. Dr. Wang gently pulled the corner of the patient's mouth lightly, found that the patient's lips were dry, and asked the nurse to apply lip oil, so as not to cause discomfort in the examination process. During the examination, it was found that 36 had a large area of metal filling on the mesial proximal surface, deep caries in the distal proximal surface, no response to the cold test, percussion pain (++), tooth mobility (I°). A soft mass was seen on the buccal side about 5 mm from the gingival margin. Press lightly to find a sense of fluctuation, and pus would overflow after the puncture with the surface anesthesia. A wide and deep periodontal pocket was detected on the buccal side, and root furcation was detected, and which periodontal depth was nearly 10 mm. 35, 37: no caries, percussion pain (−), cold test with normal control teeth, no tooth mobility. A resin-filled body was found at the surface of 46, with a feeling of pulling and roughness at the edge. The cold test was the same as the normal control tooth and no tooth mobility. A large area of metal filling was found on the surface at 16. A resin filling body was found near the center 21, and the food impaction was found near the center, percussion pain (−), no reaction on cold test, no tooth mobility. 38 and 48 existed with no jaw teeth. The oral hygiene was general. Gingival was slightly red and swollen, and bleeding was detected. After the examination, Dr. Wang informed Ms. Qin about the situation. After communication, he advised the patient to take an X-ray as the ancillary examination. The patient is cooperative. Ms. Qin's anxiety significantly reduced, and she also informed the doctor that there was no discomfort during the examination and expressed her trust to the doctor and nurse.

Then Dr. Wang arranged a nurse to accompany Ms. Qin to take the radiographic examination (Figure 11).

Patient information	Actions to take
Inference/Assumption	Question to study

第二幕

10分钟后，覃阿姨拍片回到诊位，王医生开始与患者沟通该患牙的情况"医生，这个牙还能留吗？"覃阿姨着急地问。

王医生开始跟患者解释治疗计划。

患者表示理解，并知情同意治疗。

"医生，那能麻烦您帮我看看其他牙齿吗？需要治疗的就一起治吧。"

王医生继续跟患者讲述其他牙齿情况及相关建议。临走前再次嘱咐患者，不用过多焦虑，安心休息，这些都是口腔科常见病，治疗后一般可以缓解症状。有什么问题及时打电话咨询，写下科室电话并用笔重点标注。

患者资料	拟实施治疗计划
推断 / 假设	拟学习的问题

Act II

Ten minutes later, Ms. Qin returned to the clinic. Dr. Wang began to communicate with her about the situation of the affected teeth.

"Doctor, can this tooth be saved?" Ms. Qin asked anxiously.

Dr. Wang began to explain the treatment plan. Ms. Qin showed understanding and informed consent to the treatment.

"Doctor, could you please examine other teeth? Treat them together if necessary."

Dr. Wang continued to talk to Ms. Qin about other dental conditions and related suggestions. Before leaving, Dr. Wang told Ms. Qin not to worry too much, and to rest at ease. These were common diseases in stomatology, and the symptoms could generally be relieved after treatment. If she had any problems, call for consultation in time. Dr. Wang wrote down the department phone number and marked it with a pen.

Patient information	Actions to take
Inference/Assumption	Question to study

编者：孔媛媛

译者：谭国忠

第三章
牙体硬组织非龋性疾病

第一节 牙齿"腰"上的缺口

教学目标

掌握

楔状缺损的临床表现、诊断和治疗原则。

熟悉

楔状缺损的病因。

了解

楔状缺损的发病机制。

能力目标

通过本案例学习，培养学生对楔状缺损基本知识的理解能力，理论联系实际，为临床诊治打好基础。通过学习楔状缺损的发病影响因素的相关研究，培养学生科研思维，鼓励学生探索楔状缺损的新型治疗方法。

课程思政

从楔状缺损的病因出发教会学生引导患者培养正确口腔护理方法，帮助患者预防和解决病痛，培养高尚的医德与情操。

课程设计

1. 学生8～10人为1组，通过案例情景表演、知识点汇总PPT汇报、组间讨论提问的形式进行学习。2名学生制作汇报PPT，2名学生搜集文献资料。2名学生分别饰演医生和患者，对案例进行模拟情景演绎（15分钟）。1名学生以PPT汇报的形式总结本章节知识点（10分钟）。随后教师及全体学生对情景演绎、PPT汇报的知识点进行讨论，提出问题。1名学生负责归纳总结，回答提问，教师提出指导意见（15分钟）。

2. 课后作业：各小组情景演绎剧本（考查学生对案例中，医患沟通、问诊、检查、治疗等方面的理解）；各小组提交汇报PPT（考查学生对本章节知识点的理解，学习思路）；每名学生提交楔状缺损病因–临床表现–检查诊断要点–治疗方式选择思路图（考查学生对本章节理论知识的理解，强化课堂讨论结果）。

3. 评价方式：各小组提交演绎剧本、汇报PPT，结合课堂演绎、讲解效果评分（演绎剧本占比20%，PPT占比30%）；每人提交楔状缺损诊疗思路图，根据思维完整度、对本疾病理解程度、对患者人文关怀等方面进行评价（占比50%）。

案例简介

患者因为刷牙时牙齿酸痛不适前来就诊，医生检查发现患者并没有明显蛀牙，而是在牙齿颈部发现了很深的缺损。这种缺损是导致患者出现酸痛症状的病因，案例主要围绕楔状缺损的定义、病因、临床表现、诊断要点以及治疗方法的选择展开讨论。使学生能够对楔状缺损的病因有全面的掌握，同时掌握楔状缺损的治疗方案选择。并针对楔状缺损的病因、预防方法进行讨论。

关键词

楔状缺损，酸蚀，非正中咬合力，刷牙方式，牙龈退缩，牙本质敏感

第一幕

　　52岁的李阿姨来到口腔医院看病，挂了张医生的号，张医生热情地接待了她。

　　李阿姨："张医生你好。最近1周，刷牙的时候右边牙齿酸得要命，帮我看看是怎么回事吧。"

　　张医生："好的，您可以详细描述一下具体是怎样不舒服吗？"

　　李阿姨："其实我牙齿不舒服有好几年了，以前刷牙时牙齿也会有点不舒服，但我也一直没有在意。没想到1周前我早上用冷水刷牙，牙齿酸得受不了。我赶紧对着镜子看，一看吓我一跳，右边的牙中间好像破了一个大缺口。"

　　张医生给李阿姨做了初步的检查，发现李阿姨的全口卫生状况一般，13唇侧和14、15、16、44、45颊侧牙龈退缩，探诊深度2mm，颊侧牙颈部有明显的缺损，牙本质暴露。于是张医生又问道："您平常喜欢吃硬东西吗？"

　　李阿姨："是啊，坚果、排骨这些硬硬的我都喜欢吃。"

　　张医生："您平时吃酸的东西多不多，或者会不会经常有胃反酸的症状？"

　　李阿姨："这个倒没有。"

　　张医生："您平常是怎么刷牙的呢，是竖着刷还是横着刷？"

　　李阿姨："横着刷呀，我很注意保护自己牙齿的，每天都刷牙两次，我刷得可认真了，每次都使劲刷得干干净净。"

　　张医生："您平常除了用冷水刷牙，其他时候有没有出现酸痛的情况？"

　　李阿姨："有啊，我吃冷的东西时牙齿就会酸痛难忍，而且我上次照镜子看牙齿的时候，吸了一口冷气，牙齿就特别酸痛。"

　　张医生："好的，我再给您进一步检查一下。"说着，用探针对患牙13—16、44—46逐一进行探诊，每颗患牙均出现探诊敏感的反应。

　　随后张医生测试了对照牙36，李阿姨没有感觉明显不适。随后测试患牙46，冰棒刚刚触到李阿姨的牙齿表面，李阿姨就非常痛苦地皱起眉头。

　　张医生迅速移走了冰棒并用干棉球擦干了患牙46的颊面。

　　张医生："您现在感觉怎么样，还有没有觉得不舒服？"

李阿姨："不冰了，感觉就舒服了。"

张医生随后对右侧患牙进行了冷测，反应均与46相同。

李阿姨："医生，我的牙齿为什么会变成这样啊？"

张医生："多方面的原因导致牙齿靠近牙龈那里出现了缺损，结果牙齿对外界的刺激就会很敏感，比如您的刷牙方式不对，长期横刷牙造成磨损，现在需要补牙，把缺口的部位补起来，这样才能减轻症状。"

李阿姨："好的，只要能让我不难受了就可以。"

随后，张医生向李阿姨详细说明了本次的治疗费用、治疗预后，以及预防保护措施等。

在李阿姨知情同意后，张医生为李阿姨进行了充填治疗。

张医生："牙齿补好了，您现在感觉怎么样？"

李阿姨："刚才补牙的时候牙齿还有点酸痛，现在好多了。"

张医生："好的，您回去先观察一下牙齿的情况。以后注意不要再横刷牙了，不要吃太硬的或太酸的食物。另外，如果牙齿痛了要及时回来复诊。"

李阿姨："好的，非常感谢您。"

张医生："不客气，再见！"

患者资料	拟实施治疗计划
推断 / 假设	拟学习的问题

Act I

Ms. Li, 52, came to the dental hospital for a visit based on a previous appointment with Dr.Zhang.

"Hello, Dr. Zhang. My right tooth has been sore when I brush my teeth since last week, Could you please have a look over it?" Ms. Li said.

"OK, can you describe exactly how uncomfortable it is?" Dr. Zhang asked.

"Actually, my teeth have been uncomfortable for several years, and I used to feel a little uncomfortable when I brushed them, but I never cared. One week ago, I brushed my teeth with cold water in the morning, and my teeth were so sore that I couldn't stand it. I looked in the mirror and was startled to see that there was a big gap in the middle of my right tooth." Ms. Li said.

Dr. Zhang gave Ms. Li a preliminary examination and found that Ms. Li's overall mouth hygiene was not bad. 13 labial gingival and 14, 15, 16, 44, 45 buccal gingival receded, the probing depth was 2 mm, significant defect in the cervical portion of the buccal side of the tooth, and dentin was exposed. "Do you usually like to eat hard food?" Dr. Zhang asked.

"Yeah, I like to eat hard nuts and ribs." Ms. Li answered.

"Do you usually eat a lot of sour food, or do you often experience acid reflux symptoms?" Dr. Zhang asked.

"No." Ms. Li answered.

"How do you usually brush your teeth, vertically or horizontally?" Dr. Zhang asked.

"I brush horizontally. I pay a lot of attention to protecting my teeth. I brush my teeth twice a day. I brush them very carefully, and I brush them hard and clean every time." Ms. Li answered.

"Do you usually experience any soreness in addition to brushing your teeth with cold water?" Dr. Zhang asked.

"Yes, my teeth get sore when I eat cold food, and the last time I looked at my teeth in the mirror, I took a breath of cold air and my teeth were extremely sore." Ms. Li answered.

"OK, I will give you a further examination." Dr. Zhang said. Soon after that, the affected 13–16, 44–46 were probed one by one with the probe, and each of the affected teeth showed a sensitive response.

Dr. Zhang then tested the control tooth 36, and Ms. Li didn't feel any significant discomfort. The affected tooth 46 was then tested, and the popsicle just touched the surface of Ms. Li's tooth, and Ms. Li frowned in great pain.

Dr. Zhang quickly removed the popsicle and dried the buccal surface of the affected tooth 46 with a dry cotton ball.

"How are you feeling now? Do you still feel any discomfort?" Dr. Zhang asked.

"I feel comfortable without popsicle." Ms. Li answered.

Dr. Zhang then performed a cold test on the right affected tooth, and the responses were all the same as those of 46.

"Doctor, why did my teeth turn out like this?" Ms. Li asked.

"There are various reasons in the oral cavity that cause the defects in the teeth near the gums. As a result, the teeth become sensitive to external stimuli. For example, your incorrect brushing style and long-term horizontal brushing will cause wear and tear. It is necessary to fill the teeth and patch up the chipped areas so as to alleviate such symptoms." Dr. Zhang said.

"OK, as long as it keeps me from feeling worse." Ms. Li said.

Then, Ms. Li carefully inquired about the cost of this treatment, the prognosis of treatment, and future preventive and protective measures.

Dr. Zhang then performed the restorative treatment for Ms. Li.

"The tooth is filled. How do you feel now?" Dr. Zhang asked.

"The tooth was still a little sore during the therapy, but it's much better now." Ms. Li answered.

"OK, go back and observe the condition of your teeth first. You should be careful not to brush your teeth sideways again and not to eat food that are too hard or too sour. Also, come back for a follow-up visit if your teeth hurt." Dr. Zhang said.

"Thank you very much." Ms. Li replied.

"You're welcome, bye!" Dr. Zhang said.

Patient information	Actions to take
Inference/Assumption	Question to study

编者：涂欣冉 杨 莉

译者：梁梓添

第二节　不受重视的牙齿酸软

教学目标

掌握

牙本质敏感的临床表现、诊断和常用的治疗方法。

熟悉

牙本质敏感的病因。

了解

牙本质敏感可能的发生机制及最新进展。

能力目标

通过本案例学习，培养学生对牙本质敏感的疾病基本知识的理解，理论联系实际，为口腔科普宣传打好基础。牙本质敏感的发生机制是牙体牙髓病学领域的一个未解之谜，通过这一课程让学生学习如何发现问题、思考问题、查阅资料、提出新问题、设计实验方案等科研思维，鼓励学生进行科学研究，提升自主学习能力。

课程思政

结合案例，培养学生对疾病发病的关注，特别是对特殊人群的人文关怀，培养学生拥有作为口腔医生的使命感。

课程设计

1. 课前学生8～10人为1组分配任务，阅读案例后提出问题，以问题为导向方式列出学习重点，查找资料，课前文献阅读4学时，课上案例讨论2学时（其中脑力激荡10分钟、问题列举5分钟、讨论及引导50分钟、总结15分钟）。本案例是希望学生能由"牙齿酸软"开始讨论，涉及的知识点有：牙本质敏感的定义、鉴别诊断、病因及危险因素。尤其是磨损、磨耗、酸蚀、应力集中、唾液这些非龋性危险因素在牙本质敏感的发生和发展中所起的作用。在此案例中教师应引导学生重点讨论牙本质敏感常见的非龋性因素，涉及的龋性因素引导学生区分，不做重点讨论。

2. 课后作业：预习并准备第二幕讨论，做"牙本质敏感的病因及危险因素"的思维导图。

3. 评价方式：课上表现占70%、作业占30%。课上表现使用自评、组内及组间互评、教师评价表评分（教师评价包括纪律性、参与度、组内影响力、团队合作力、协调能力等方面）。

关键词

牙本质敏感，酸蚀，磨损，磨耗，流体动力学说，脱敏治疗

案例简介

本案例学习牙本质敏感相关内容，设计分为两幕进行。

第一幕主要讨论牙本质敏感的定义、牙本质敏感的病因及危险因素。牙本质敏感是一种症状，很多疾病都伴随这种症状，通过学习和讨论，让学生知道什么情况才能诊断为牙本质敏感，以及牙本质敏感与龋病、非龋性疾病的关系。牙本质敏感重在预防，且要想获得良好的远期治疗效果，需要尽可能地找出病因及危险因素并对其进行干预。因此，第一幕的重点和难点为牙本质敏感致病病因和危险因素分析，为此提供多篇参考文献进行阅读。

第二幕主要讨论牙本质敏感可能的发生机制、治疗原理和方法。牙本质敏感的发生机制是个未解之谜，目前仍是牙体牙髓病学的研究热点之一。教师应了解目前的研究进展，激发学生们对研究产生兴趣，了解研究的过程，比如发现问题、查阅文献、总结目前研究状况和待解决问题、设计课题、进行实验、发表文献等过程。接下来再讨论牙本质敏感的治疗原理、常见的脱敏成分、临床的治疗方法及效果。最后模拟临床接诊牙本质敏感患者的过程，重新复习牙本质敏感所有的知识点，加深对牙本质敏感的病因及危险因素、预防和治疗方法的理解。

第一幕

　　25岁的吴小姐特别爱喝冰镇饮料，但近1个多月来自觉喝冰镇饮料时牙齿出现酸软，自行使用脱敏牙膏刷牙仍无好转，于是就诊于口腔医院，想查明牙齿酸软的原因并对其进行治疗。

　　临床检查发现（图12），其口内多颗牙齿唇颊侧颈部存在牙龈退缩和牙本质暴露，后牙𬌗面部分釉质缺损，冷测时出现牙本质敏感。经病史询问，患者存在用力刷牙、爱吃硬食、酸性食物和饮用饮料等不良习惯，存在夜磨牙的现象，平时偶有反酸、"烧心"等身体不适，无高血压、糖尿病、心脏病等其他系统性疾病。

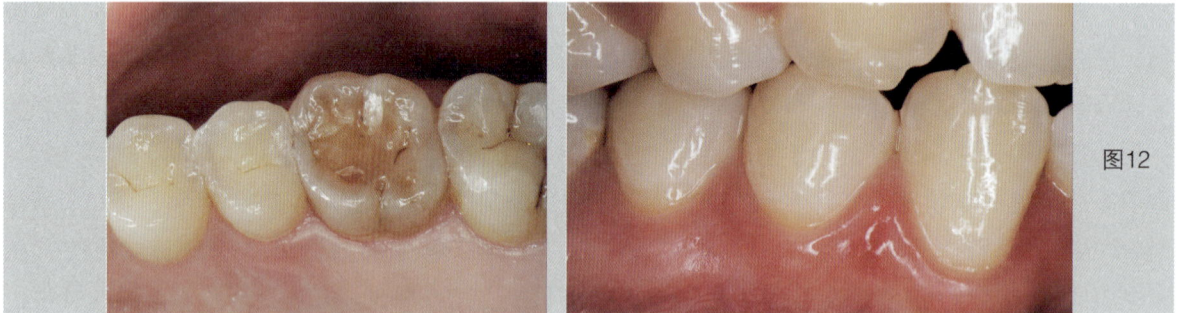

图12

患者资料	拟实施治疗计划
推断 / 假设	拟学习的问题

Act I

Ms. Wu, 25 years old, loves to drink cold drinks, but in the past few months or so, she felt that her teeth were sore and soft when she drank cold drinks. She brushed her teeth with desensitizing toothpaste but without improvement, so she visited a dental hospital to find out the cause of her sore and soft teeth and get treatment.

Clinical examination revealed (Figure 12) that many teeth had gingival recession and dentin exposure on the labial and buccal sides of the cervical, partial enamel defects on the occlusal surface of the posterior teeth, and dentinal hypersensitivity on the cold test. Upon historical inquiry, Ms. Wu had bad habits such as vigorous brushing, being addicted to hard foods, acidic foods and beverages, grinding teeth at night, and occasional physical discomforts such as acid reflux and heartburn, but had no other systemic diseases such as hypertension, diabetes mellitus, or heart disease.

Patient information	Actions to take
Inference/Assumption	Question to study

第二幕

　　医生向患者解释了病情，对出现敏感的牙齿进行了诊室脱敏治疗，嘱咐患者配合家庭脱敏治疗，并要改正不良刷牙及饮食习惯，建议诊治夜磨牙及胃肠疾病。

患者资料	拟实施治疗计划
推断 / 假设	拟学习的问题

Act II

The doctor explained the patient's condition, performed in-office desensitization treatment for the sensitive teeth, instructed the patient to cooperate with home desensitization treatment and to correct bad brushing and eating habits, and suggested diagnosis and treatment of night grinding and gastrointestinal diseases.

Patient information	Actions to take
Inference/Assumption	Question to study

编者：蔡冬萍

译者：梁梓添

第三节 磨损

教学目标

掌握

1. 磨损的发病原因。

2. 磨损的临床表现。

3. 磨损的预防及治疗方法。

熟悉

1. 根据磨损的发病原因及患者年龄的不同，合理选择治疗方案。

2. 磨损的发病原因及影响因素。

了解

1. 磨损治疗后的饮食方式、口腔卫生的健康宣教。

2. 磨损的发病率；磨损在不同（年龄、职业、饮食习惯）人群中发病率的区别。

能力目标

通过本案例学习，加深对磨损的理解，由于课本知识量较少，拓展知识面需提高学生查阅、筛选及阅读国内外文献的能力。通过思维导图或其他形式整理碎片知识，提高通过图文的表现方式展示学习成果的能力。

课程思政

1. 培养正确的爱伤观念。

2. 应用循证医学的方法制订治疗方案。

3. 磨损治疗后饮食方式、口腔卫生的健康宣教。

课程设计

1. 课程内学生随机分组或自由结合，8～10人为1组，每组成员任务分配如下：收集资料、查阅文献、制作思维导图、汇总问题制作PPT。以磨损、楔状缺损为主要症状的鉴别诊断，磨损的影像学特点、治疗原则为主要学习目标。重点内容讨论时间约占70%，其余内容讨论时间约占30%。

2. 课后作业：讨论结束后1周内每人需交1篇小组讨论记录，由组长收齐送交指导教师。

3. 评价方式：课上表现占70%、作业占30%。课上表现使用自评、组内及组间互评、教师评价表评分（教师评价包括纪律性、参与度、组内影响力、团队合作力、协调能力等方面）。

案例简介

通过讲述牙齿磨损的患者来就诊时的情景、介绍患者的基本信息，了解患者的病情。使学生不仅了解了病例的背景，也学习问诊的方式、方法，在细节里体现医生应有的人文关怀。

本案例的设计分为两幕进行。

第一幕学生由"磨损的表现"开始讨论，在此幕中教师引导学生重点讨论磨损的发生、诊断、鉴别诊断、临床表现、并发症及其与磨耗的区别。颞下颌关节紊乱与磨损的相互关系不是本次重点，避免学生讨论过于深入。

第二幕针对"磨损的治疗"展开讨论，熟悉牙体牙髓的治疗方案并拓展讨论修复、正畸、颞下颌关节的相关治疗，教师需把握讨论的深度和广度。

关键词

磨损，磨耗，脱敏，牙本质

第一幕

65岁的戴维在女儿的陪同下来口腔医院看病，挂了科室号以后，在诊室外排队等候。

10分钟后，戴维先生被分配到李医生的诊室。

李医生："戴维先生，我有什么能帮到您的吗？"

戴维："我20多岁的时候，就开始感觉前面上下牙隐隐地不舒服。当时去补过一次牙，很不舒服。后来我一直未看过牙医。"

李医生："现在口腔技术发展很迅速，不会像以前一样了。您是有什么不适吗？可以跟我描述一下，或者需要我帮您解决什么问题？"

戴维："我前面下排牙齿越来越短，吃冷的热的都很酸痛。"

李医生："其余还有什么不舒服吗？"

戴维："经常塞牙，吃饭就塞牙。其他牙牙根和牙龈之间有小小的缝隙。"

李医生："这些缝隙痛吗，酸吗？"

戴维："不痛不酸，就很小的缝隙，不仔细看也发现不了，我掉了几颗牙，待会儿你可以看到。"

李医生："好的，那让我来检查一下，看看您的牙齿都有什么问题。"

戴维："好的医生，您轻一点！"

李医生："好的，您放心。如果感到不舒服，您举左手，我就立刻停止。"

李医生为戴维进行口腔检查，患者对刃𬌗。上下前牙牙冠变短，咬合呈面状接触，磨牙𬌗面呈光滑平面，釉质边缘锐利。𬌗曲线变平滑。15、35、45缺失，11、14、23、24、31、32、41、42、44、46、47牙颈部缺损，46𬌗面见金属充填体。颞下颌关节未见明显异常。

李医生："您平时经常磨牙吗？"

戴维："是的，前牙总感觉不舒服，磨一磨牙齿就舒服了。"

李医生："有夜磨牙的习惯吗？"

戴维："有，老毛病了。"

李医生："这样有多久了，治疗过吗？"

戴维："有20年了，没有治疗过。"

李医生："牙齿现在有什么不适吗？"

戴维："对冷热很敏感，不吃冷热的食物就不会不舒服。"

李医生："刷牙方法也不对，您刷牙是不是打横刷了？"

戴维："是啊，我们那个年代都是这么刷的。"

李医生："好的，您先跟我的助手护士小张学习一下正确的刷牙方法，以及牙刷、牙膏、饮食习惯的选择，我把牙齿情况记录一下，做一个治疗方案给您。"

护士小张拿出水平颤动拂刷法的示意图，为戴维进行示范。

患者资料	拟实施治疗计划
推断／假设	拟学习的问题

Act I

David, 65 years old, came to the dental hospital accompanied by his daughter and waited in line outside the office after registration.

10 minutes later, David was assigned to Dr. Li's office.

"David, how can I help you?" Dr. Li asked.

"When I was in my twenties, I started to feel discomfort in my upper and lower front teeth. I went for a filling at that time and it was very uncomfortable. I have never visited the dentist since then." David said.

"Nowadays, dental technology is developing very fast, so it won't be the same as before. Do you have any discomfort that you can describe to me, or what can I do for you?" Dr. Li said.

"My lower front teeth are getting shorter and shorter, and it feels sore when I eat cold or hot food." David said.

"Anything else?" Dr. Li asked.

"The front teeth are often clogged, and I get stuffed when I eat. There are small gaps between the roots of the other teeth and the gums." David replied.

"Do these gaps hurt? Are they sore?" Dr. Li asked.

"It doesn't hurt or cause sores. It's just a minimal gap. You can't find it unless you look carefully. I lost a few teeth, and you can see it later." David replied.

"OK, then let me check what's wrong with your teeth." Dr. Li said.

"OK doctor, please be gentle!" David said.

Dr. Li said to David, "OK, don't worry. If there is any discomfort you can raise your left hand and I will stop immediately."

Dr. Li performed an oral examination for David, and David had a crossbite. The crowns of the upper and lower anterior teeth became shorter, the occlusion was in faceted contact, the jaw surface was smooth and flat, and the enamel margin was sharp. The jaw curve became smooth. 15, 35 and 45 were missing. 11, 14, 23, 24, 31, 32, 41, 42, 44, 46 and 47 were cervically defected, and 46 had metal fillings on the jaw surface. No significant abnormalities were seen in the temporomandibular joint.

"Do you usually like to grind your teeth?" Dr. Li asked.

"Yes, the front teeth always feel uncomfortable, and grinding the teeth makes me feel better." David answered.

"Do you have the habit of grinding your teeth at night?" Dr. Li asked.

"Yeah, it's been a long time." David answered.

"How long has this been going on, have you had it treated?" Dr. Li answered.

"For 20 years without treatment." David answered.

"Do you have any discomfort with your teeth now?" Dr. Li asked.

"My teeth are very sensitive to the hot and cold, but I won't feel uncomfortable if I don't eat the hot or cold." David answered.

"It seems that the way you brush your teeth is incorrect. Did you brush your teeth horizontally?" Dr. Li asked.

"Yes, that was how I did in those days." David answered.

"OK. Firstly, you should learn the correct way to brush your teeth with my assistant nurse Xiao Zhang, as well as the choice of toothbrushes, toothpaste, and eating habits. I will record the dental situation and make a treatment plan for you." Dr. Li said.

Xiao Zhang took out the diagram of the modified bass method and demonstrated it to David.

Patient information	Actions to take
Inference/Assumption	Question to study

第二幕

在助手护士的帮助下戴维学会了正确的刷牙方法并树立了良好的口腔卫生习惯。经过口腔状况评估后，李医生建议：

1. 患者前牙磨损较重，建议患者可针对敏感的症状对症治疗，考虑患者年龄较大，建议择期分次充填楔状缺损。

2. 可以佩戴功能𬌗垫改善夜磨牙状况。

3. 如患者全身状况合适并且经济条件支持，可以考虑进行咬合重建。

患者资料	拟实施治疗计划
推断 / 假设	拟学习的问题

Act II

With the help of Xiao Zhang, David learned the correct way to brush his teeth and established good oral hygiene habits. After the oral condition assessment, Dr. Li recommended that:

1. The patient's anterior teeth are heavily worn, and it is suggested that the patient can be treated symptomatically for the symptoms of sensitivity. Considering the patient's age, the wedge-shaped defect is recommended to be filled in stages.

2. Functional jaw pads can be worn to improve the condition of nocturnal grinding teeth.

3. If the patient's general condition and family economy permit, occlusal reconstruction can be considered.

Patient information	Actions to take
Inference/Assumption	Question to study

编者：吴　磊

译者：梁梓添

第四节　牙齿的"隐形杀手"

掌握

牙隐裂的概念、临床表现、诊断、治疗原则。

熟悉

牙隐裂的病因。

了解

国际牙裂综合征分类方法。

能力目标

通过本案例学习，学生要掌握牙隐裂的病因、临床表现、诊断、治疗方法和预后判断。本案例从"咬合痛"出发，启发学生结合病史，考虑都可能是哪些疾病，应进行哪些检查。思考不同检查结果所对应的治疗方案及预后，提高学生临床思辨能力。

课程思政

牙隐裂的诊断需细致、耐心地进行患牙排查，需培养学生高度的临床责任感。牙隐裂的预后不确定性高，需提升学生病情告知技巧、提醒学生注意事项。

课程设计

1. 课前学生8～10人为1组分配任务，阅读案例后提出问题，以问题为导向列出学习重点，查找资料，课前文献阅读4学时，课上案例讨论2学时（其中脑力激荡10分钟、问题列举5分钟、讨论及引导50分钟、总结15分钟）。希望学生能由"咬合痛"开始讨论，涉及的知识点有：牙隐裂的病因、临床表现、诊断、治疗方法和预后判断。在此案例中教师应引导学生重点讨论牙隐裂的病因和治疗方法的选择。涉及的其他牙裂类型，比如牙根纵裂，引导学生区分类型即可，不做重点讨论。

2. 课后作业：预习并准备第二幕讨论，做"咬合痛"接诊流程的思维导图。

3. 评价方式：课上表现占70%、作业占30%。课上表现使用自评、组内及组间互评、教师评价表评分（教师评价包括纪律性、参与度、组内影响力、团队合作力、协调能力等方面）。

案例简介

一位因"咬合痛"就诊的患者，接诊医生发现其26近中邻猞面深窝沟，越过边缘嵴，告知患者治疗方案，患者表示考虑。1周后，该患者因咬硬物，牙齿出现剧烈自发痛，再次就诊，接诊医生检查后给予了适当治疗。

本案例分为两幕进行。

第一幕希望学生从"咬合痛"出发，结合病史，考虑都可能是哪些疾病，应进行哪些检查。

第二幕随着病情的发展，希望学生思考不同检查结果所对应的治疗方案及预后。通过回答本案例提出的问题，掌握牙隐裂的病因、临床表现、诊断、治疗方法和预后判断。

关键词

牙隐裂，咬合痛，咬诊，咬合创伤

第一幕

　　某周日下午，50岁的陈先生来口腔医院看病，导诊护士在询问患者病情及病史后让其等待。半小时后，陈先生坐在了张医生的治疗椅上。

　　张医生："您好，请问您牙齿怎么不舒服呢？"

　　陈先生："我最近吃东西时觉得牙齿酸。"

　　张医生："请问是哪边牙齿呢？"

　　陈先生："就是左上侧大牙，你看看是什么问题呢？"

　　张医生："好，一会儿我帮您检查一下。您最近是觉得咬东西牙齿痛呢，还是觉得咬东西无力呢？"

　　陈先生："也不是痛，也不是没力，就是酸软，你知道吧？"

　　张医生："那您是每次一咬到东西就觉得不舒服，还是吃着吃着才开始不舒服呢，或者是吃到什么特定的东西，比如冷的、甜的，才感觉不舒服呢？"

　　陈先生："也不是每次都痛，原来就是吃甘蔗什么的有时候会觉得酸软，上星期就感觉有点加重了，不知道咬到哪里会突然痛一下，痛了就不敢再咬了，跟冷热好像没有什么关系，你说能是什么问题呢？"

　　张医生："好，您先放松一点，我来检查一下。"

　　张医生仔细地为陈先生进行了检查，发现26骀面近中窝沟深，形态如图13所示，探诊患处略酸痛不适。其余牙未见明显龋坏及缺损。牙龈色粉，质韧，未探及明显牙周袋。

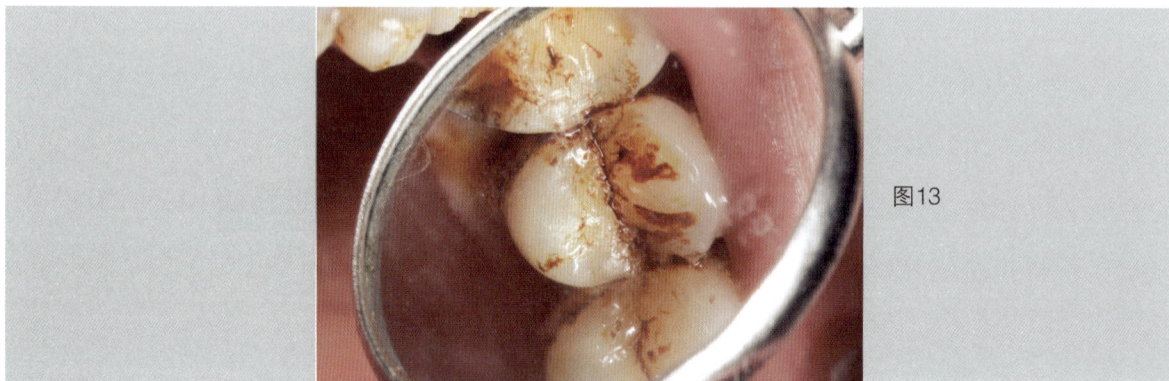

图13

　　张医生："先生，您左上倒数第二颗牙齿上面有一条裂纹，每次咬到裂纹的时候就会觉得痛。"

　　陈先生忙问："裂纹？为什么会有裂纹呢？"

　　张医生："牙齿出现裂纹的原因有很多，主要还是由外力造成的。比如，您喜欢咬一些不好咬的东西，像甘蔗之类的，牙齿就容易裂。"

　　陈先生："我倒是挺喜欢吃甘蔗，天天都吃，以后不能吃了吗？这牙还能嚼东西吗？"

　　陈先生看着张医生，期待医生可以拯救他没有甘蔗的日子。

患者资料	拟实施治疗计划
推断 / 假设	拟学习的问题

Act I

One Sunday afternoon, Mr. Chen, 50 years old, came to the dental hospital to visit a dentist. Half an hour later, Mr. Chen sat in Dr. Zhang's dental chair.

"Hello, what's wrong with your teeth?" Dr. Zhang asked.

"My teeth feel sour when I eat recently." Mr. Chen answered.

"Which side of the tooth is it?" Dr. Zhang asked.

"It's the molar on the upper left side. What's the problem?" Mr. Chen said.

"OK, I will check it for you later. Do you feel pain or lack of strength when you bite recently?" Dr. Zhang asked.

"It's not painful or weak. It's just sour, you know." Mr. Chen said.

"Do you feel uncomfortable every time you bite into something, or do you feel uncomfortable only when you eat something, or do you feel uncomfortable only when you eat something specific, such as something cold or sweet?" Dr. Zhang asked.

"Not every time. I don't dare to bite again. It doesn't seem to have anything to do with heat or cold." Mr. Chen answered.

"OK." Dr. Zhang said.

Dr. Zhang examined carefully and found that the mesial fossa and groove of 26 were deep in the occlusal surface, and the shape was as shown in the Figure 13. The affected area was slightly sore and uncomfortable after probing. No obvious caries or defects were found in other teeth. Gingiva was pink and tough, and no obvious periodontal pocket could be seen.

"Mr. Chen, there is a crack on the penultimate tooth on the upper left. You feel pain every time you bite into the crack." Dr. Zhang said.

Mr. Chen hurriedly asked, "Crack? Why?"

"There are many reasons for teeth cracks, mainly external forces. For example, if you like to bite on something hard, such as sugar cane, your teeth are easy to crack." Dr. Zhang replied.

"I really like to eat sugar cane and eat it every day. Can't I eat it anymore? Is this tooth still useful?" Mr. Chen asked.

Patient information	Actions to take
Inference/Assumption	Question to study

第二幕

张医生："通过目前检查来看，您现在暂时还没有牙神经发炎的症状，也就是说裂纹不算太深，可以先试着保守治疗。首先要把这颗牙齿磨低一点儿，降低它受到的咬合力。然后要把这颗牙套住，减少吃东西时这颗牙向外爆开的力。"

陈先生："怎么套住呢？"

张医生："可以做一个临时牙冠保护，观察一段时间，如果症状消失，再换成永久的牙冠。"

陈先生："还有可能症状不消失吗？那怎么办？"

张医生："如果症状加重，出现牙神经痛，就要先摘除牙神经，再做牙冠。"

陈先生："我感觉没那么严重啊，现在也是偶尔痛，注意一点也可以吃东西的。我先考虑一下吧，回去商量一下，有空了我再来。"

张医生："可以的，您回去跟家人商量一下，我把病情写在病历里，忘了可以看一下。牙齿裂开这种问题还是要尽快治疗，不然越裂越深，最后可能需要拔牙。回去不要再咬硬的东西了。"

陈先生："好的，我尽量。"

1周后，患者陈先生再次出现在诊室。

陈先生："张医生啊，我昨天吃饭时，饭里有颗沙子，一下就咯到我这颗牙上了，痛得我一晚都没睡，不会这么快就裂大了，要拔牙了吧？"

张医生："我先给您检查一下，好吧？昨晚痛的时候有没有吃止痛药啊？"

陈先生："没有，就想早上赶紧过来看一下。"

张医生对陈先生进行了仔细地检查，告知患者病情、治疗方法及预后。陈先生表示非常后悔上次没有接受治疗，并接受了本次的治疗方案。

患者资料	拟实施治疗计划
推断 / 假设	拟学习的问题

Act II

"According to the current inspection, you have no symptoms of inflammation of the pulp, which means that the crack is not too deep, so you can try conservative treatment first. The first step is to grind the tooth a little lower so as to reduce the force of the bite. The tooth should then be braced to reduce the force of the tooth popping out when eating." Dr. Zhang said.

"How to get it braced?" Mr. Chen asked.

"You can have a temporary crown and observe it. If the symptoms disappear, you can replace it with a permanent crown." Dr. Zhang replied.

"What if symptoms don't disappear?" Mr. Chen asked.

"If the symptoms worsen and there is pain in the nerve, the nerve should be removed first and then the tooth crown should be made again." Dr. Zhang replied.

"I don't think it is that severe. It hurts occasionally now. I can still eat if I am careful. I'll think about it first, and then discuss it with my family. I'll come back when I am available." Mr. Chen said.

"No problem. You can go back to discuss with your family. I will note the condition in the medical record. Take a look if you forget. The problem of cracked teeth should be treated as soon as possible, otherwise the cracks will get deeper and deeper, and eventually the teeth may need to be extracted. Go back and don't bite anything hard." Dr. Zhang replied.

"OK." Mr. Chen said.

A week later, Mr. Chen returned to the clinic again.

"Dr. Zhang, I had a grain of sand in my meal yesterday, and it hit my tooth. It hurt so much that I didn't sleep all night. The crack can't be so big that the teeth should be pulled out, right?" Mr. Chen asked.

"Let me check it first, OK? Did you take painkillers when it hurt last night?" Dr. Zhang said.

"No, I just want to come and have a look in the morning." Mr. Chen replied.

Dr. Zhang examined Mr. Chen carefully and informed him of his condition, treatment and prognosis. Mr. Chen expressed his regret for not receiving treatment last time and accepted the treatment plan this time.

Patient information	Actions to take
Inference/Assumption	Question to study

编者：王一舟

译者：谭国忠

第五节 都是牙尖惹的祸

教学目标

掌握

1. 畸形中央尖的定义。
2. 畸形中央尖的好发部位及临床表现。
3. 畸形中央尖的临床特点及处理原则。
4. 牙齿发育异常的主要类型。

熟悉

1. 牙齿数目异常的临床表现和治疗原则。
2. 牙齿结构异常的临床表现和治疗原则。
3. 牙齿萌出与脱落异常的临床表现和治疗原则。

了解

了解与牙齿发育异常有关的综合征。

能力目标

以畸形中央尖折断病例的诊治为中心，引出牙齿发育异常的各种概念和知识，掌握牙齿发育异常主要类型，熟悉各种牙齿发育异常的临床表现和治疗原则，培养学生发散思维和横向思维能力，能做到举一反三。同时，在查阅相关文献的过程中培养学生自主学习的意识与能力，培养学生主动参与整个学习过程，并与小组成员分工合作的能力。

课程思政

1. 畸形中央尖为异常发育，对于由此引发的牙齿疼痛家长较焦虑，医生需要有耐心、有爱心，对患者的病情及家长的焦虑与担忧感同身受，体现人文关怀。

2. 对畸形中央尖早期干预可以降低并发症的发生，应强调定期口腔检查的重要性。对于口腔疾病，我们应当防患于未然！

课程设计

1. 学生10~12人为1组，提前2周给学生发放案例及相应参考文献，用于预习案例，查阅牙齿发育异常相关文献，分析案例。课上共4学时，其中第一幕讨论共2学时，小组成员分析、讨论案例，提出问题，以问题为导向进行讨论，列出学习目标问题（课上阅读分析案例10分钟、小组内讨论案例30分钟、小组合作总结目标问题40分钟）。第二幕讨论共2学时，回顾案例10分钟、讨论及解决目标问题20分钟、分组汇报两幕目标问题答案40分钟、案例总结反馈10分钟。第一幕重点学习牙齿形态异常相关知识，引导学生重点讨论畸形中央尖的定义、好发部位、临床表现及处理原则，牙齿形态异常的主要类型及临床表现。第二幕给学生提供患者X线片，讨论畸形中央尖折断引起年轻恒牙牙髓感染的处理方法，引导学生掌握牙髓再生治疗的适应证，同时引导学生熟悉牙齿结构异常、牙齿数目异常、牙齿萌出与脱落异常的临床表现和诊治原则，让学生不要混淆各类牙齿发育异常的概念。由于本章节各部分内容比较独立、零散，最后让学生通过PPT汇报和思维导图串联牙齿发育异常整个章节的内容。

2. 课后作业：第一次课程结束后作业为将第一幕牙齿形态异常讨论总结的目标问题答案制作PPT或思维导图，预习并准备第二幕讨论。第二次课程结束后作业为制作PPT或思维导图串联及总结牙齿发育异常整个章节的内容。

3. 评价方式：课上表现占70%、作业占30%。课上表现使用学生自评、组内互评、教师评价表评分（教师评价表主要包含学习态度、课堂参与度、课堂能力评价、沟通与合作技巧等方面）。

案例简介

本案例学习牙齿发育异常相关内容，设计分为两幕进行。

第一幕通过畸形中央尖折断的案例引出本章节的主题——牙齿形态异常，引导学生重点讨论畸形中央尖的定义、好发部位及临床表现，牙齿形态异常的主要类型及临床表现，同时提供相关参考文献，通过讨论引导学生熟悉各类牙齿形态异常的诊断及处理原则。

第二幕给学生提供X线片，通过讨论畸形中央尖折断引起年轻恒牙牙髓感染的处理方法，引出牙髓再生治疗的概念，掌握其适应证，同时需要引导学生熟悉牙齿结构异常、牙齿数目异常、牙齿萌出与脱落异常的临床表现和诊治原则，让学生不要混淆各类牙齿发育异常的概念。

关键词

畸形中央尖，牙齿形态异常，牙齿结构异常，牙齿数目异常，牙齿萌出与脱落异常

第一幕

一天下午，表情痛苦的童童由焦虑的妈妈带到口腔医院儿童口腔科就诊。

童童妈妈："您好！我女儿牙齿痛，我预约了王医生的号看牙。"

导诊："好的，请您稍等一下。（分诊）请您带小孩到2诊室王医生处就诊。"

穿着朴素的妈妈领着一位穿着校服、乖巧的小女孩走进了诊室。

童童妈妈问："请问您是王医生吗？"

王医生："是的，我是王医生，请问我有什么可以帮到您？"

童童妈妈："王医生您好！这是我女儿童童，她最近2周牙齿痛，吃东西更痛，都不敢咬东西，您看看是什么问题？"

王医生："好的，童童你把书包给妈妈拿着，坐到牙椅上，阿姨帮你检查一下牙齿。"

童童乖巧地坐到牙椅上，时不时地用手捂着右脸。

王医生："童童，你今年几岁？你哪边牙齿痛？"

童童小声地回答："医生，我今年11岁半，我右边下面的牙齿痛。"

王医生："你这边牙齿痛大概有多久？"

童童："上个月吃东西的时候就不舒服，我没有和妈妈说，这2周痛得比较厉害才和妈妈讲。"

王医生开始仔细检查童童的牙齿（图14），发现童童的口腔卫生良好，牙齿刷得很干净。但是45殆面中央见一圆环状折裂痕，探诊无反应，叩诊（＋），无松动，牙髓温度测试：冷测无反应；34、35、44殆面中央窝处可见一圆锥形的牙尖，有少量磨损，探诊（－）、叩诊（－）、无松动，冷测正常反应，牙龈未见异常；余牙未见异常。

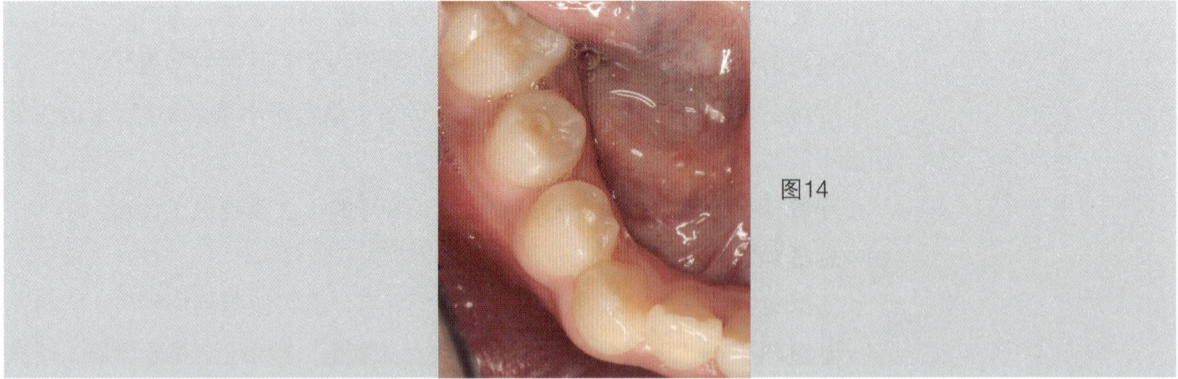

图14

患者资料	拟实施治疗计划
推断 / 假设	拟学习的问题

Act I

One afternoon, a girl named Tongtong with a painful expression was taken to the Department of pediatric stomatology of the Stomatological Hospital by her anxious mother.

"Hello, my daughter has a toothache. I had an appointment with Dr. Wang." Tongtong's mother said.

"OK, please wait a second." the guide replied.

"Please take your child to see Dr. Wang in clinic 2." the triage said.

Tongtong's mother, dressed in plain clothes, led a well-behaved little girl in a school uniform into the clinic room.

"Are you Dr. Wang?" Tongtong's mother asked.

"Yes, I'm Dr. Wang. What can I do for you?" Dr. Wang said.

"Hello, Dr. Wang. This is my daughter, Tongtong. She had a toothache in the last two weeks. It's even more painful to eat. She doesn't dare to bite anything. What's the problem?" Tongtong's mother replied.

"OK, Tongtong, give your schoolbag to your mother and sit on the dental chair. I will help check your teeth." Dr. Wang said.

Tongtong sat quietly on the dental chair and covered her right face with her hand from time to time.

"Tongtong, how old are you? Which side of your tooth hurts?" Dr. Wang asked.

Tongtong answered in a low voice, "Doctor, I am 11 and a half years old, and I have a toothache on the lower right side."

"How long have you been suffering from this toothache?" Dr. Wang asked.

"I felt uncomfortable when I ate last month. I didn't tell my mother. I only told my mother that the pain had worsened in the past two weeks." Tongtong answered.

Dr. Wang began to examine Tongtong's teeth carefully (Figure 14) and found that Tongtong's oral hygiene was good and her teeth were clean. However, a circular fracture could be seen in the center of 45 occlusal surface, probing pain (–), percussion pain (+), no obvious tooth mobility, pulp vitality test: no response on cold test; a conical cusp could be seen in the central fossa of the occlusal surface of 34, 35 and 44, with a small amount of abrasion, probing pain (–), percussion pain (–), no obvious tooth mobility, normal response to cold test, no abnormality in gingiva; no abnormality in other teeth.

Patient information	Actions to take
Inference/Assumption	Question to study

第二幕

　　王医生检查完童童的牙齿后，让童童妈妈带童童去放射科拍摄X线片。X线片示：45发育至Nolla分期8期，根管口呈喇叭口状，根尖周可见低密度影像，牙周膜间隙增宽（图15）。王医生告知牙齿的诊断为：45慢性根尖周炎；34、35、44畸形中央尖，并告知童童妈妈牙齿的治疗方案、费用及预后，童童妈妈知情同意，并签署了治疗同意书。

　　最后童童妈妈感叹道，都是畸形牙尖惹的祸，要是早点带童童看牙医就好了！

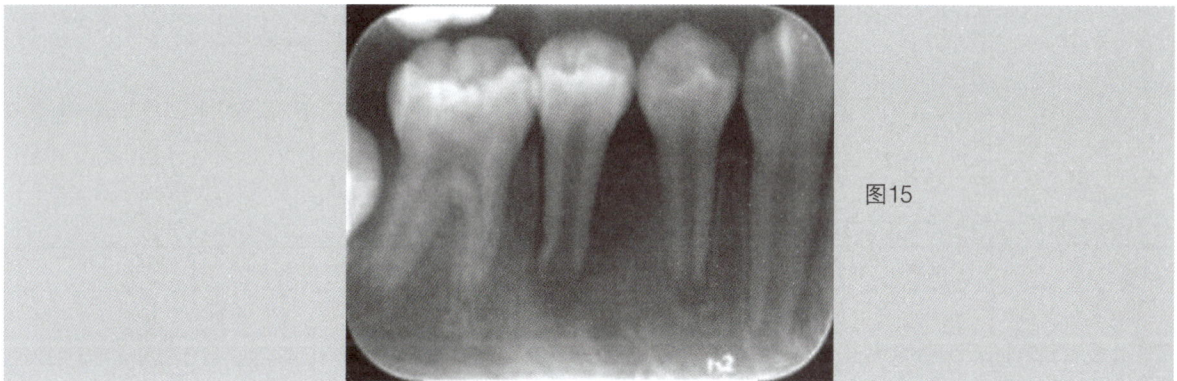

图15

患者资料	拟实施治疗计划
推断 / 假设	拟学习的问题

Act II

After examining Tongtong's teeth, Dr. Wang asked Tongtong's mother to take Tongtong to the radiology department to take an X-ray. The results of the radiographic examination were as follows: 45 developed to Nolla 8 stage, the root canal foramen was bell-mouthed, the periapical low-density image was seen, and the periodontal ligament space was widened (Figure 15). Dr. Wang informed the diagnosis of the tooth: 45 chronic periapical periodontitis; 34, 35, 44 central cusp, and informed Tongtong's mother of the treatment plan, the cost and the prognosis of the tooth. Tongtong's mother gave informed consent and signed the treatment consent.

Finally, Tongtong's mother sighed that it was all the fault of the malformed cusps. If only she had taken Tongtong to visit a dentist earlier!

Patient information	Actions to take
Inference/Assumption	Question to study

编者：曾素娟　方　颖
译者：刘珍妮　陈　彦

第六节 "白牙星人"历险记

教学目标

掌握

1. 儿童牙外伤的分类。
2. 儿童牙外伤的临床检查及注意事项。
3. 儿童恒牙外伤的治疗原则。
4. 牙髓切断术的适应证。

熟悉

儿童恒牙外伤病史采集时如何体现良好的医患沟通能力及人文关怀。

了解

1. 儿童牙外伤的发病情况。
2. 儿童恒牙外伤的危害和预防。
3. 牙外伤的追踪和预后评估。

能力目标

培养学生以儿童牙外伤病例诊治为中心的临床思维能力,掌握儿童牙外伤的分类、临床表现及诊治原则。在学习过程中查阅牙外伤最新治疗指南,了解牙外伤研究最新研究进展,培养学生检索文献、查阅文献及整理文献的能力。在学习讨论牙外伤过程中,以学生为主导,培养其提出牙外伤相关问题、分析问题、解决问题的能力,并提高学生的团队合作能力。

课程思政

在接诊牙外伤儿童患者的过程中,首先需要关注全身情况,比如是否有需要紧急处理的全身性问题,再关注牙齿的情况;且牙外伤的预后与转归具有很不确定性,需要用发展变化的眼光看待问题。外伤后儿童及家长可能处于极度紧张和焦虑的状态,不仅需要解释清楚牙外伤的治疗方案及可能的预后,也需要在诊疗过程中对患儿及家长做好安抚工作。因为涉及第三方的赔偿等,临床病历具有法律效力,所以临床医生需要按照实际情况详细进行病历书写。

课程设计

1. 课前学生以10～12人为1组，提前1周发放案例及相应参考文献，课堂提出问题，以问题为导向的方式列出学习重点。共6学时，第一幕课堂分析、讨论案例2学时（课堂上阅读分析案例情景10分钟、讨论案例30分钟、汇总问题30分钟，教师就课堂讨论内容、学生表现情况做总结10分钟）。在第一幕中，希望学生根据不完整的病案提出问题，分析、归纳出必须了解的牙外伤的流行情况，巩固年轻恒牙的概念，年轻恒牙牙根发育的相关知识以及由此带出的一系列牙外伤病史采集中需要注意的相关问题。第二幕讨论共2学时（回顾案例10分钟、讨论案例30分钟、汇总问题30分钟，教师就课堂讨论内容、学生表现情况做总结10分钟）。在第二幕中，希望学生根据完整的临床检查，建立牙外伤接诊的临床思维（包括牙外伤临床检查注意事项、各牙外伤的治疗原则、相似临床表现的牙外伤类型的鉴别诊断）。每幕结束后小组组长归纳总结目标问题，各组员针对小组学生的课堂表现进行评价。第三幕主要回顾第一幕及第二幕学习目标，根据第一幕、第二幕总结归纳的目标问题，以小组形式进行小组学习成果汇报，汇报以PPT、文献汇报、病例汇报等形式进行。课堂分析、讨论案例2学时（回顾案例5分钟，分组汇报并讨论两幕目标问题答案70分钟，本章节内容总结5分钟）。

2. 课后作业：第一次课后，学生通过查找文献、专著、课本、网络资源等学习资料回答目标问题，形成自己的主张，归纳做成PPT、思维导图或word文档等。第二次课后，根据案例所给资料，学生自己归纳出主诉、现病史、既往史等内容，制订本案例牙外伤类型的治疗计划，并书写1份临床病历。第三次课，学生课上成果汇报，课后1周内以word文档或PPT串联牙外伤章节知识并发送给教师。

3. 评价方式：课上评价占70%、作业形式占30%。课上评价主要包括学生相互评价表、自我评价表、教师评价表等相结合的形成性评价。教师评价表主要包含学习态度、课堂能力评价、沟通与合作技巧等内容。

案例简介

8岁男孩小明在与同学玩耍时不慎跌倒，致上前牙折断。经过医生检查发现，小明的右上前牙冠折露髓，需要进行治疗。牙外伤常伴有牙体牙髓组织和牙周组织损伤，预后存在不确定性，后期若炎症控制不佳，出现牙髓坏死、牙根吸收等情况可能需要拔除患牙。

本案例的设计分为三幕进行。

第一幕提供情景，教师引导学生对案例进行分析、讨论，找出本案例所涉及的年轻恒牙外伤理论部分的知识。本幕重点引导学生掌握牙外伤的分类、儿童恒牙外伤的好发年龄及牙位、儿童恒牙外伤断冠的保存方式，熟悉医患沟通及医疗纠纷等知识。

第二幕提供完整的病史资料和患儿的口内照、根尖片，但不包含诊断，让学生针对病例资料提出本案例的诊断及治疗原则。本幕重点引导学生掌握儿童恒牙外伤的临床表现、临床检查、注意事项、临床诊断及治疗原则。

第三幕提供病例诊断及治疗方案。本幕重点引导学生掌握牙髓切断术的适应证，了解儿童恒牙外伤的危害、预后评估及预防，最后结合案例让学生讨论本案例的治疗方案是否合理。

通过此案例的学习，引导学生掌握儿童恒牙外伤的分类、临床表现、临床检查、注意事项、临床诊断及治疗原则，熟悉医患沟通及医疗纠纷等知识，了解牙外伤的危害、预后评估及预防。

关键词

儿童恒牙外伤，牙髓切断术，断冠粘接术，序列治疗

第一幕

　　早上10点，小明妈妈在田里种地，邻居跑来对小明妈妈说："小明妈，小明老师来电话说小明摔倒了，你快去看看吧！"小明妈妈不急不慢地说："摔倒了怕什么，小孩子磕磕碰碰很正常。"邻居说："好像把牙齿撞断了，还流血呢！你快去看看。"小明妈妈说："他都8岁了，我家孩子可没你家孩子娇气，再说学校里还有老师，等我干完这点儿活就去。"

　　中午，小明妈妈赶到学校，看见小明嘴里咬了块棉花，眼睛哭得通红。小明妈妈赶紧问老师怎么回事，老师说："小明在走廊和同学玩，不小心摔倒，把牙齿摔断了。校医已经检查过，应该没事，止血就行了，反正牙齿总要换的。"小明这时还是觉得痛，小明妈妈着急地说，"快点去医院吧，不能总是痛啊！"

　　赶到医院已经是下午2点了。

　　医生拉着小明的手问："什么时候摔倒的呢？在哪儿摔倒的？是怎么摔倒的？"

　　小明说："我在走廊和同学玩耍，后面有同学突然把我推倒了。"

　　医生问："你疼不疼啊？摔断的牙齿在哪里呢？"

　　小明说痛，老师赶忙说："摔断的牙齿在这，我怕弄脏，特意用纸巾包着带来了。"

　　医生解释道："小明的牙齿属于牙外伤，而且是恒牙，是不会再换的牙齿，需要及时治疗，争取最佳治疗时机，小明来得还算及时，但是效果不能肯定，一般外伤的牙齿治疗后还需要密切观察，预后不佳的话不排除有拔牙的可能。"

　　小明妈妈听到医生这样讲，当场大哭。她没想到事情这么严重，孩子小小年纪就可能需要拔掉一颗要伴随自己一辈子的恒牙。

患者资料	拟实施治疗计划
推断 / 假设	拟学习的问题

Act I

At 10 a.m., Xiaoming's mother was farming in the field. The neighbor ran to Xiaoming's mother and said, "Xiaoming's mother, Xiaoming's teacher called and said that Xiaoming fell down. Go and have a look!" Xiaoming's mother said calmly, "It doesn't matter. It is normal for children to fall over." The neighbor said, "It seems that his tooth is broken and is still bleeding! You should go to have a look." Xiaoming's mother said: "He is 8 years old now. My child is not as delicate as yours. Besides, there are teachers at school. I will go when I finish this work."

At noon, Xiaoming's mother rushed to school and saw Xiaoming was biting a piece of cotton in his mouth, and his eyes were red with tears. Xiaoming's mother asked the teacher what had happened. The teacher said, "Xiaoming was playing with his classmates in the corridor, and accidentally fell down and broke his tooth. The school doctor has already checked it. It should be fine. Anyway, his teeth will be replaced soon." Xiaoming still felt pain at this moment. Xiaoming's mother said anxiously, "Let's go to the hospital immediately, or it will be pain continuously!"

It was already two o'clock in the afternoon when they arrived at the hospital.

The doctor took Xiaoming's hand and asked, "When and where did you fall down? How did you fall down?"

"I was playing with my classmates in the corridor, and some classmates suddenly pushed me down." Xiaoming answered.

"Does it hurt? Where is the broken tooth?" the doctor asked.

Xiaoming said he was in great pain, and the teacher said, "The broken tooth is here. I was afraid that it would get dirty. I specially wrapped it with tissue."

"It's a kind of tooth trauma, and the tooth is a permanent tooth, which will not be replaced again. They need timely treatment and strive for the best treatment effect. Although Xiaoming went to the hospital in time, the effect of treatment is uncertain. Generally, traumatic teeth need to be closely observed after treatment. If the prognosis is poor, the tooth may be extracted." the doctor explained.

Xiaoming's mother cried when she heard what the doctor said. She never realized the situation was so severe that Xiaoming might need to have a permanent tooth pulled out at an early age.

Patient information	Actions to take
Inference/Assumption	Question to study

第二幕

医生对小明进行了仔细的病史询问和口腔检查，否认头晕、呕吐等情况，否认全身系统疾病及药物过敏史。

口外检查可见患者颌面部对称，开口型、开口度正常，口内检查（图16）见11切端斜形折裂，余留牙体组织唇侧位于龈上4mm，腭侧位于龈上约2mm，牙髓暴露，露髓孔直径约2mm，叩诊（+），无松动，龈沟局部渗血，未探及深牙周袋；21牙体组织未见明显缺损，叩诊（+），无松动，牙龈未见异常，未探及牙周袋；12部分萌出，12、53、63牙体组织未见异常，叩诊（-），无松动，牙龈未见异常；62牙体组织未见异常，叩诊（-），Ⅱ°松动，牙龈未见异常。余牙未见明显异常。根尖片显示：11冠部低密度暗影及髓，根管内未见高密度充填影像，牙根发育达Nolla分期8期，根尖周未见低密度暗影；21未见明显牙体缺损，牙周膜未见异常，根尖周未见低密度暗影；62牙根吸收2/3；12、22发育达Nolla分期8期。

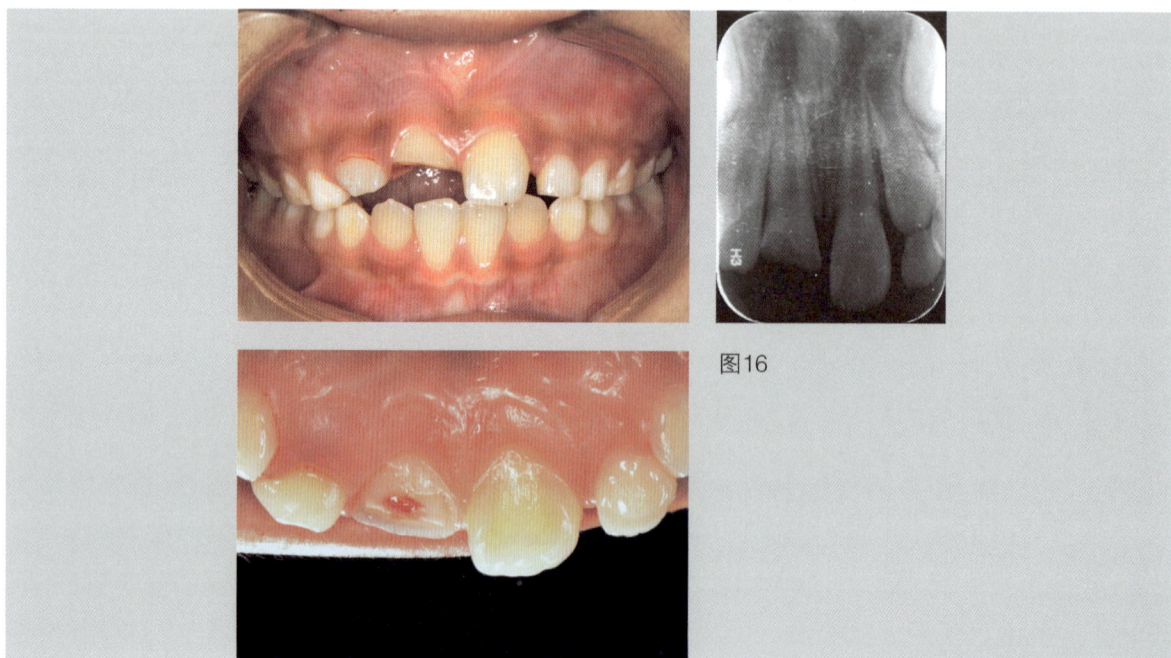

图16

患者资料	拟实施治疗计划
推断 / 假设	拟学习的问题

Act Ⅱ

The doctor carefully inquired about Xiaoming's medical history and conducted an oral examination. Xiaoming denied dizziness and vomiting, without a history of systemic diseases or drug allergy.

Extraoral examination showed that the maxillofacial region of the patient was symmetrical, with normal open–mouth type and degree, while intraoral examination (Figure 16) showed that 11 cutting ends were oblique fractures. The labial side of the remaining tooth tissue was located 4 mm above the gingiva, and the palatal side was located about 2 mm above the gingiva. The dental pulp was exposed, the diameter of the pulp hole was about 2 mm, percussion pain (+), no obvious tooth mobility, local bleeding in the gingival sulcus, and no deep periodontal pocket was detected. No obvious defect, percussion pain (+), no obvious tooth mobility, no abnormality in gingiva and no periodontal pocket were found in 21; 12 partial eruption, 12, 53, 63 tissue no abnormality, percussion pain (–), no obvious tooth mobility, gingival no abnormality; No abnormality, percussion pain (–), tooth mobility (Ⅱ°), and no abnormality in gingiva were found in 62. No obvious abnormality was found in the remaining teeth. Apical radiographs showed: 11 radiolucent shadows in crowns and no radiopaque filling images in pulp and root canals. Root development reached Nolla stage 8, and no radiolucent shadows were found around tooth apices; 21 no obvious tooth defect, no abnormality of periodontal ligament and no radiolucent shadow around apical region were found. The root resorption of 62 reached 2/3 of the whole root; the development of 12 and 22 reached Nolla stage 8.

Patient information	Actions to take
Inference/Assumption	Question to study

第三幕

　　本案例患者的临床诊断为：11复杂冠折；21牙震荡。治疗方案为与患者家长沟通拟行11冠髓切断术+断冠粘接术；21定期复查。患者家长签署知情同意书。

　　术后1个月复查，患者自诉患牙无不适，检查患牙充填物完好，叩诊无不适。X线片示：11、21根尖区未见异常。

患者资料	拟实施治疗计划
推断 / 假设	拟学习的问题

Act Ⅲ

The clinical diagnosis of this case was as follows: 11 complicated crown fractures, 21 tooth concussions. After communicating with the patient's parents, the treatment plan was to perform 11 crown pulpotomy+reattachment of crown fragment; 21 periodic review. The patient's parents signed informed consent.

One month after the operation, the patient claimed that there was no discomfort in the affected teeth. The fillings in the affected teeth were intact, and there was no discomfort on percussion. The X-ray showed that there was no abnormality in the apical area of 11 and 21.

Patient information	Actions to take
Inference/Assumption	Question to study

编者：曾素娟　封　琼　方　颖　盛　婷
译者：刘珍妮　陈　彦